THE SOUTH BEACH DIET

200 Easy Solutions for Everyday Meals

SUPER QUICK COOKBOOK

Arthur Agatston, MD

Author of the #1 *New York Times* Bestseller *The South Beach Diet*

RODALE

© 2010 by Arthur Agatston, MD
The South Beach Diet® is a Registered Trademark of the SBD Trademark Limited Partnership.
Photographs © 2010 by Ben Fink

Rodale books may be purchased for business or promotional use or for special sales. For information, please write to: Special Markets Department, Rodale Inc., 733 Third Avenue, New York, NY 10017.

Printed in the United States of America

Book design by Christina Gaugler
Food styling by Megan Schlow
Prop styling by Dani Fisher

ISBN-13: 978–1–60529–333–2 hardcover

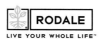

We inspire and enable people to improve their lives and the world around them

For busy families everywhere

who have made cooking and eating healthy food

a way of life

And for Sari, Evan, and Adam

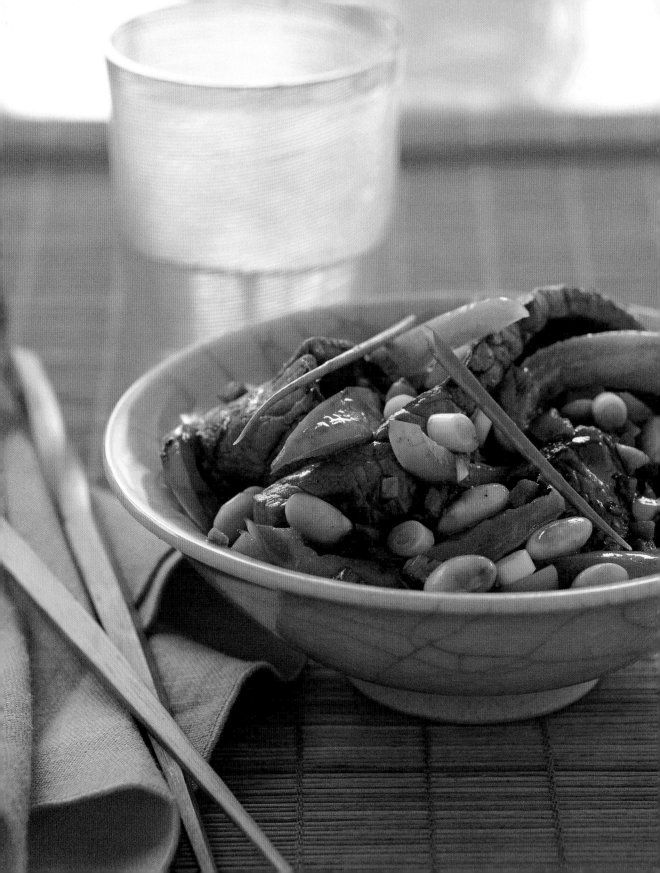

CONTENTS

ACKNOWLEDGMENTS

This healthy, time-saving cookbook could not have been produced without the combined efforts of a great team of associates.

First I would like to thank Maria Rodale for her support and for always believing in our mission of changing the way America eats. Others at Rodale who provided their time and expertise include publisher Karen Rinaldi, publishing director Pam Krauss, executive art director Amy King, book designer Christina Gaugler, test kitchen director JoAnn Brader, and senior production editor Nancy N. Bailey.

The absolutely delicious and healthy recipes in the book could not have been achieved without two of the best recipe developers in the business, Sandra Rose Gluck and Kate Slate. And I also want to acknowledge the invaluable contributions from SouthBeachDiet.com and from devoted members of the Web site's Century Club. A very personal thanks to Bonnee Binker, for allowing us to use one of her (and my) favorite recipes, the Black Bean Brownies, on page 245. And, for the beautiful color photographs, my appreciation goes to photographer Ben Fink, food stylist Megan Schlow, and prop stylist Dani Fisher.

On the South Beach Diet side, as always, kudos to my director of nutrition, Marie Almon, for her recipe ideas, meal plans, and attention to the little details that make these recipes work, and to my editorial director, Marya Dalrymple, for her essential writing and editing skills. I also want to thank Margo Lowry of the South Beach Diet partnership, for the idea for the Two-Mushroom Cauliflower Soup recipe, on page 69, and executive assistant, Marcia Collado, whose expertise at the keyboard helped get this book off the ground. Thanks, too, to my agent, Mel Berger, and our publicists Sandi Mendelson and Cathy Gruhn of Hilsinger-Mendelson for their constant support.

And last, but hardly least, there would be no book without my wife and partner, Sari Agatston, whose firm belief in my passion to stop heart disease and in the South Beach Diet lifestyle has helped us reach so many of you today.

COOK QUICKLY, EAT SLOWLY

For many busy people, "home cooking" has come to mean a take-out meal from the closest fast-food franchise. In fact, recent statistics show that the average American household spends about $2,500 annually at take-out establishments and restaurants, or about 71 percent of what it spends on groceries ($3,500). This percentage is even higher for householders aged 25 to 34 (81 percent) and for people who live alone (79 percent). And these numbers appear to be growing—along with our waistlines.

The sad reality is that two-thirds of the adults and one-third of the children in this country are either overweight or obese. Today, the typical baby boomer male weighs just shy of 200 pounds and the average female weighs more than 170. That's in part because a typical fast-food quarter-pound cheeseburger packs a hefty 500 calories, the large fries another 500, the supersized soda 300 more, and an ice cream dessert an additional 500. That's 1,800 calories from a single meal! Couple that with the fact that most people don't exercise enough and it's small wonder that conditions like diabetes and heart disease are on the rise, and few of us feel very good about what we see in the mirror.

Not a very appetizing way to start off a cookbook, is it? But I bring up these statistics for a good reason. If we continue at this sad pace, dining out more than we're eating in and skipping the supermarket for the drive-thru, this country's burgeoning obesity epidemic will have dire consequences, not just for our present and future health but for our health-care system as well. Doctors and hospitals simply won't be able to handle all the new cases of prediabetes, diabetes, heart disease, stroke, kidney disease, and other obesity-related conditions. The good news? One of our most effective remedies for *all* of these ailments can be found in our own refrigerators, pantries, and cupboards.

That said, I know few of us have time to linger in the kitchen, stirring up elaborate meals from scratch. As a practicing cardiologist who often gets home from the office late and who doesn't cook all that well himself, I rely on my very busy wife to make sure I eat nutritious meals. Fortunately, she also stocks the kitchen with the kind of healthy ingredients needed to put good meals together quickly. So when she isn't home to cook due to her own busy schedule, I can put together an easy, speedy meal.

As this book will show you, if you plan your meals ahead, shop thoughtfully, and organize your pantry and kitchen for quick cooking, you'll easily be able to turn out healthy, delicious food for the whole family with very little stress. And I guarantee you'll look and feel better for it, too.

I often like to remind my patients who enjoy cooking that preparing a meal quickly should *not* translate to rushing at the table. Eating thoughtfully and slowly, really tasting what we eat, allows us to experience a sense of fullness naturally without overeating. I remember as a child always being told to clean my plate. For me, that was an invitation to wolf down dinner and get on to other things. Today, I'm sorry to say that I still tend to eat a bit too quickly; I often have to remind myself not to take second helpings before my brain gets the signal that I'm full.

On the South Beach Diet, you won't leave the table hungry, but you shouldn't feel stuffed, either. I like to say that you should eat until you are satisfied, not until you are full. Research now shows that routinely galloping through meals often leads to chronic overeating and obesity. This is because putting too much food in your stomach too quickly can interfere with the body's feedback mechanisms, allowing you to continue to take in more calories because you don't yet feel full. I recommend starting lunch or dinner with a filling cup of soup, like the White Bean and Escarole Soup with Shaved Parmesan on page 62, or with a fiber-rich salad like the Fennel, Cucumber, and Watercress Salad on page 219. I also suggest putting down your fork between bites. Don't worry if you leave some food on your plate; if you are satisfied, you've had enough. And please, enjoy a few bites of a decadent dessert from time to time. (My favorite, Chocolate Truffle Tartlets, is on page 232.)

Preparing the healthy, superquick recipes in this book represents the ultimate win-win scenario: Not only will you be eating far better than you would were you spending your food dollars in restaurants or on processed foods, but the time you save in the kitchen means that you will have more time to relax, savor your food, and enjoy some good conversation with family and friends. And as far as I'm concerned, that's what home cooking should be about.

—*Arthur Agatston, MD*

QUICK, DELICIOUS, AND NUTRITIOUS EATING ON THE SOUTH BEACH DIET

The South Beach Diet is a lifestyle that allows you to enjoy a wide variety of nutritious foods—including nutrient-dense, high-fiber carbohydrates (vegetables, fruits, legumes, whole grains), lean protein (fish, poultry, lean cuts of beef), low-fat dairy, and good fats (olive oil, canola oil)—as you lose weight or maintain a healthy weight. And the good news is that all of these foods lend themselves to quick and easy meals the whole family can enjoy.

Ever since our *South Beach Diet Quick & Easy Cookbook* was published in 2005, fans of the diet have been asking for even more healthy recipes that can be prepared in 30 minutes or less. The more quick recipes you have in your repertoire, the easier it is to incorporate good, nutritious meals into the day's activities—and you'll have more time to spend reading, playing with your kids, or meeting friends for a fun outing.

Today, it's even easier than it was 5 years ago to turn out healthful meals in a snap, thanks in part to the dazzling array of already-prepped ingredients available in most supermarkets. While you'll probably pay a bit more for pre-washed salad blends, prediced fruits and vegetables, and grated cheeses, for many cooks the time savings these ingredients offer is worth the premium price. Of course the right kitchen equipment makes cooking quicker and easier too. We describe some of our favorite time-saving gear on page 12.

Whatever phase of the South Beach Diet you're on, with this book you'll never be at a loss for what to prepare, whether it's a quick breakfast or snack, a speedy entrée, or a fast (and healthy) dessert. And to inspire you further, on pages 14 to 21 we've included suggestions for Grab-and-Go dishes to take on the road or to the office; Dishes for Two that are just right when it's just the two of you (or even just yourself); and some No-Cook Salads for those really insane days.

You'll find that the biggest trick to quick cooking isn't a trick at all. Preparing truly "fast food" basically boils down to thinking ahead. Not only will advance planning save you time and energy, it will put dollars in your pocket as you shop smart with your grocery list in hand. To help you get started, we've provided 2 weeks of Meal Plans for both Phase 1 and Phase 2, using many of the recipes in this book (see pages 268 and 283). Follow these plans to the letter or use them as guidelines, mixing and matching our recipes with your family's healthy favorites, depending on the occasion, your tastes, and what's seasonal at the market.

And by the way, don't forget to ask for some help when it comes time to get dinner on the table. Invite your spouse into the kitchen to wield the knives and wash the dishes, but also try to include the kids. Studies show that children are more interested in eating healthy foods if they've helped to prepare them, and that the earlier they get comfortable using a whisk or wooden spoon, the better. Let them measure dry ingredients, crack the eggs, or peel a carrot. As they get better at these tasks, you'll be surprised at how much time you save when they work by your side.

HOW TO USE THIS BOOK

We recommend skimming through the book first to get inspired by the mouthwatering recipes and colorful photos. The book starts with quick breakfasts; continues with appetizers, soups, salads, main dishes, and desserts; and ends with more complicated make-ahead dishes that take extra time for chilling, stewing, or baking—but provide big time-saving dividends in the end. For lighter meals, there is a chapter of Main-Dish Salads (page 79), and for the non-meat-eaters or those trying to cut back on meat, a chapter of Meatless Mains (page 185), including some vegan options. Not only will cooking meatless once or twice a week save you money (meat is one of the most expensive items on a grocery bill), but decreasing your intake of saturated fats and increasing your intake of fiber and cell-protective antioxidants is good for you.

As you look at the specific recipes (and the Meal Plans on pages 268 and 283), do so with an eye to what phase of the diet you're on. If you're on Phase 1, for example, you'll be avoiding refined starches and sugars, but you'll still find plenty of satisfying recipes in every chapter, including taste-tempting desserts. And once you're on Phase 2 or Phase 3, you can, of course, enjoy all the recipes in the book (the phase designations are clearly indicated). Each recipe also features Hands-On Time (the active time you spend in the kitchen chopping, stirring, seasoning, and so on) and Total Time (how long it takes to make a dish from start to finish). Some recipes lend themselves to repurposing, and leftovers can be transformed into entirely new dishes later in the week. You'll see these "Cook Once, Eat Twice" suggestions throughout the book. In addition, if a recipe is *so* superquick that it can be prepared in 15 minutes or less, you'll see a little clock icon to indicate this.

Whatever recipes you choose, we suggest that you read them carefully up front and make sure you have all the ingredients and pots and pans out and ready before you begin. Many of our recipes are quick sautés or stir-fries that come together in just a few minutes; you don't want to be hunting for a second nonstick skillet or the jar of oregano once you've got things going. Some cooks find that doing some of this organizing in the morning saves time and energy later in the day. Others like to do their prepping days in advance, chopping and freezing vegetables, fruits, and other foods for future use (for more on this, see page 9). Whether you're an "advance prepper" or not, always pay attention to the "meanwhiles" in the recipes. Doing two things at once, like chopping the basil while you're steaming the sugar snap peas, is key to getting food on the table fast.

The Phases: A Quick Review

For those new to the diet, here's a crash course on the fundamentals of the South Beach Diet's three phases. For complete information on the diet, look for Dr. Agatston's *The South Beach Diet Supercharged* or visit SouthBeachDiet.com.

Phase 1: This is the shortest and strictest phase of the diet, which lasts for just 2 weeks. Phase 1 is for people who have a substantial amount of weight to lose or experience strong cravings for sugary foods and refined starches. During this phase, you'll jump-start your weight loss and stabilize your blood sugar levels to minimize cravings by eating a diet based on healthy lean protein (fish and shellfish, chicken and turkey, lean cuts of meat, soy); loads of vegetables and plenty of salads; beans and other legumes; nuts; reduced-fat cheeses; eggs; low-fat dairy; and good unsaturated fats, such as extra-virgin olive oil and canola oil. You'll enjoy three satisfying meals a day plus two snacks, and you'll even be able to have some dessert. What you won't be eating are starches (bread, pasta, rice) or sugars (including fruits and fruit juices). While this may be hard at first, your cravings will soon disappear and in just 2 weeks you'll be adding many of these foods back into your life. Exercise during this and all of the phases of the diet is important to your overall health and will improve your results.

Phase 2: Those who have 10 pounds or less to lose, who don't have problems with cravings, or who simply want to improve their health can start the diet with Phase 2. If you're moving on to Phase 2 from Phase 1, you'll find that your weight will continue to drop steadily (although more slowly) and your cravings will have subsided. You'll gradually reintroduce many of the foods that were off-limits on Phase 1, including more good carbohydrates, such as whole-grain breads, whole-wheat pasta, and brown rice, as well as whole fruits and some root vegetables (like sweet potatoes). You'll also be able to have a glass of red or white wine with meals if you like.

Phase 3: You'll enter this phase once you have reached your healthy weight. At this point in the diet you'll be able to monitor your body's response to particular foods easily, and you'll find yourself naturally making the right food choices most of the time. You can enjoy a decadent dessert on occasion and when you do, you will probably find you've satisfied that sweet tooth after just a few bites. By the time you enter Phase 3, the South Beach Diet will have become a way of life, and its sound eating principles will help you keep the weight off while staying fit and healthy.

SUPERQUICK, BUDGET-CONSCIOUS SHOPPING

Superquick cooking starts with efficient shopping. For many people this also means adhering to a food budget. When grocery shopping is just a mindless endeavor, you are likely to end up with a cart full of processed foods with minimal nutritional value. Instead, observe these time- and money-saving tips and shop more strategically.

Plan your meals in advance. There's nothing more frustrating and time-consuming than emergency trips to the supermarket for essentials you forgot to restock. Planning your meals a week at a time helps avoid unnecessary shopping trips and kitchen frustration. You can use the Meal Plans on pages 268 to 297 for guidance or make up your own menus based on your supermarket's specials or your family's preferences. If you're on a strict budget, think about enjoying more expensive dishes like salmon and lamb chops less frequently and focusing mostly on cheaper chicken and turkey dishes and a meatless meal or two each week. Also check out your staples and make sure you have the basics for preparing a week's worth of healthy meals. On page 7 we list many of those you'll need for the recipes in this book.

In addition, think about who you'll be feeding. Will your spouse be away on business? Are the kids involved in school activities? Have you been invited out? Is company coming for the weekend? You may need more or less food than usual, depending on the week's events. And consider what dishes could be doubled to make more than one meal (see our Cook Once, Eat Twice recommendations with various recipes throughout the book). If you do have extra food, freeze it in individual portions for those nights when you *really* don't have any time to cook, or for nights when "the cook" is away.

Make a shopping list, but be flexible. Once you've planned your menus and thought about the recipes you'd like to prepare, draft an organized shopping list. Put produce in one column; dry goods in another; meat, poultry, and fish in another. You may find it easiest to envision the layout of your usual market, creating your list aisle by aisle so you can move through the store most efficiently.

If you're a big-box-store shopper, consider whether you actually do save money by buying in bulk, or if much of that 25-pound bag of whole-wheat flour will ultimately go to waste. If you're a farmers' market shopper, think about hitting the stalls at the end of the day when vendors often cut their prices in order to avoid hauling produce back home. If you're a supermarket shopper, check the circulars so you can take advantage of the best bargains and coupons. And don't forget about shopping in ethnic markets where you can often get great buys on produce, spices, yogurt, condiments, specialty meats, and more.

Wherever you shop, take advantage of produce in season. It's healthier and cheaper, and if you freeze fruits and vegetables at their peak, you'll be well set months later.

Finally, try not to shop when you're hungry and don't stray from your list unless a great bargain beckons. Studies show that more than half of all grocery purchases are unplanned, and that's how a food budget gets out of control.

Check your receipts. How many times have you fretted in a long grocery checkout line, and then, in your rush to get out of the store, forgotten to check your receipt? Checkout errors are surprisingly frequent, so the best thing to do if you want to save dollars is watch the price of each item as it's scanned, including your coupons. Sale items in particular often come up wrong. If you think there's an error, challenge it right then. Your diligence can really add up to big bucks at the end of year.

THE SUPERQUICK PANTRY

Having a well-stocked kitchen is essential for quick, easy, and spontaneous cooking. You may not have a separate walk-in pantry, but making sure your cupboards, fridge, and freezer are well organized and stocked with often-used items is a great time-saver.

Start by assessing what's on hand if you haven't gone through your staples in quite a while. Open jars of herbs and spices and give them the sniff test; if they smell musty or don't smell at all, toss them and buy new. Also give your cooking and salad oils a taste test for rancidity. Then "go shopping" in your fridge. You may be surprised at how many half-empty jars of Dijon are hiding in there. Get rid of anything that looks ancient or suspicious or that you think you'll never use again. And finally, clean out the freezer of foods that are more than a few months old, aren't dated, or have freezer burn.

Stocking Your Pantry (and Fridge) for This Book

To save you some planning time, we've listed the staples you'll need to prepare the recipes in this book. We haven't included fresh produce, breads, or commonly used ingredients like onions and garlic, lemons, and limes, but we have included dairy, cheeses, and soy products, just so you can familiarize yourself with the types we commonly use. Remember that these are simply suggestions for what to have on hand to save time later. Ultimately, setting up a pantry depends on your personal taste and, of course, your budget. Here are the foods we consider South Beach Diet essentials:

Baking supplies. Baking powder, baking soda, bittersweet dark chocolate, semisweet chocolate chips (also mini), unsweetened dark baking chocolate, sugar-free chocolate syrup, unsweetened cocoa powder, cream of tartar, shredded and flaked unsweetened coconut, lite unsweetened coconut milk, whole-wheat pastry flour, old-fashioned rolled oats, mini phyllo shells, quinoa flakes. See also Sweeteners, on page 9.

Beans and legumes, canned. Black beans, chickpeas, lentils, pinto beans, white beans, or any other beans you love (they're interchangeable in many of the recipes). Of course, if you have some time, you can cook dried beans from scratch.

Broth, canned. Lower-sodium chicken broth and vegetable broth, clam broth. (See page 10 for a homemade chicken stock recipe to freeze for later use.)

Cheese, reduced-fat. Blue, Cheddar, feta, goat cheese, Gruyère, light spreadable cheese wedges, Mexican blend, Monterey Jack, part-skim mozzarella, part-skim ricotta, Swiss. Note: Many of the recipes in this book call for grated Parmesan. Buy regular Parmesan, either pregrated or shredded, or better yet in chunks to grate yourself. Parmigiano-Reggiano is expensive, but its rich flavor is worth the price. For maximum storage, wrap cheese first in waxed paper and then in plastic wrap. And don't be afraid to scrape the natural mold off better cheeses if it forms.

Condiments. Prepared horseradish, sugar-free apricot jam, mayonnaise, Dijon mustard, hot pepper sauce (red), jalapeño pepper sauce, red salsa, green salsa, black bean salsa, reduced-sodium soy sauce, Worcestershire sauce

Dairy. Light (1.5%) buttermilk, buttermilk powder, fat-free cottage cheese, 1% whipped cottage cheese, reduced-fat cream cheese, fat-free half-and-half, fat-free evaporated milk, fat-free milk, 1% milk, nonfat dry milk powder, light and reduced-fat sour cream, no-sugar-added lite whipped topping, nonfat and low-fat plain yogurt, nonfat (0%) plain Greek yogurt, artificially sweetened strawberry low-fat or nonfat yogurt

Extracts. Pure almond extract, pure vanilla extract

Flour and meal. Chickpea flour, whole-wheat flour, white whole-wheat flour, whole-wheat pastry flour, flaxmeal

Fruit, dried. Dried apples, pitted prunes

Grains. Quick-cooking barley, bulgur, semipearled farro, quick-cooking oats, quinoa, quick-cooking brown rice

Herbs, dried. Basil, bay leaves, fennel seeds, garlic powder, Italian herb blend, herbes de Provence, marjoram, oregano, poultry seasoning, rosemary, rubbed sage, taco seasoning, tarragon, thyme. See also Spices, below.

Nuts, nut butters, and seeds. Natural almonds, slivered almonds, cashews, flaxseed, dry-roasted peanuts, natural no-sugar-added peanut butter, pecans, pine nuts, pistachios, hulled pumpkin seeds, sesame seeds, sunflower seeds

Oils. Canola oil, cooking spray (for coating baking pans and grills only), trans-fat-free margarine (vegetable oil spread), extra-virgin olive oil, peanut oil, safflower oil, dark sesame oil, walnut oil

Pasta, whole-wheat. Angel hair (cappellini), lasagna, shells or other small shaped pasta, spaghetti

Soy products. Plain unsweetened soy milk, baked tofu, lite firm tofu, lite silken tofu, soft silken tofu, medium-firm tofu, soy nuts, TVP or TSP granules

Specialty items. Anchovy paste or canned anchovies, artichoke hearts in water, nonpareil capers, chipotle chiles in adobo, Thai red curry paste, salad-cut hearts of palm, dried mushrooms (porcini), roasted jarred peppers (halves and slices), pickled jalapeño peppers, canned tomatillos, sun-dried tomatoes (in oil and dried), water-packed light tuna (not albacore), mini whole-wheat phyllo tartlets

Spices. Adobo seasoning, ground allspice, ground cardamom, cayenne, ancho chile powder, chipotle chile powder, chili powder, chili seasoning, cinnamon (ground and whole sticks), cloves (ground and whole), ground coriander, ground cumin, curry powder, five-spice powder, garam masala, ground ginger, ground mace, ground mustard, nutmeg (ground and whole), paprika, black pepper (ground and whole peppercorns), red pepper flakes, salt (regular and kosher), turmeric

Sweeteners. Light agave nectar, granular sugar substitute. Note: The recipes in this book were tested using the granular sugar substitute Splenda (buy it in boxes or bags; do not use the packets in these recipes, since they are a different texture and sweetness). If you would prefer to try a natural sweetener such as stevia or agave nectar in certain recipes calling for granulated sugar substitute, keep in mind that these products are much sweeter than Splenda and cannot be directly substituted in a recipe. If you do try recipes using natural sweeteners, we would be interested in hearing your results.

Tomatoes, canned. Crushed tomatoes, diced tomatoes, diced tomatoes with garlic, spicy diced tomatoes, fire-roasted tomatoes, tomatoes in purée, tomato paste (buy tubes to avoid waste), no-salt-added tomato sauce

Vinegar. Balsamic vinegar (dark and white), cider vinegar, red wine vinegar, rice vinegar, sherry vinegar

Wine. Dry red wine, dry white wine

Keep in mind that storing your staples properly is the key to freshness, particularly if you don't use up items quickly. Once you get home from the market, transfer bulk herbs and spices to labeled jars and grains to airtight containers. Store olive oil and canola in a dark cupboard, and nut oils in the refrigerator. Use the freezer for perishables such as nuts, whole-wheat flour, and whole-wheat tortillas, which can go bad quickly.

Maximizing Your Freezer

Quick cooking will go even faster if you have a well-stocked, well-organized freezer. What a relief to know that there are prechopped onions and peppers in there, not to mention those fabulous fillets of wild salmon you bought on sale and a pan of Spinach and Four-Cheese Lasagna (page 257) ready for reheating. When it comes to your freezer, consider the following:

Cool it right. The ideal freezer temperature is about 0°F. Use a freezer thermometer to check. Freezers that are too warm (between 25° and 31°F) freeze food too slowly, allowing ice crystals to form and creating freezer burn.

Sari's Chicken Stock

The Agatston kitchen is never without a supply of homemade chicken stock in the freezer. This is Dr. Agatston's wife Sari's favorite recipe. It can be used in any of the recipes in this book that call for canned broth. Adding lots of celery and carrots and a piece of fresh ginger gives the broth special richness. Freeze the stock in 1-quart resealable freezer bags (freeze them flat on a baking sheet and, once frozen solid, they can be stacked for storage).

    3 pounds chicken parts, skin removed

    1 pound carrots, halved

    8 celery stalks, cut into 2-inch pieces

    1 large onion, unpeeled and quartered

    5 large garlic cloves, unpeeled

    1 (2-inch) piece fresh ginger

    5 large sprigs fresh parsley, or a handful of parsley stems (optional)

    1½ teaspoons salt

Cut a few gashes in the chicken parts. Place the chicken, carrots, celery, onion, garlic, ginger, parsley (if using), and salt in a large stockpot with about 4 quarts of cold water to cover. Bring to a boil over high heat, then immediately reduce the heat to a simmer. Cook the stock at a low simmer, skimming the foam as needed, for 2 to 2½ hours, until the stock is flavorful. Add more water if necessary to keep the chicken covered.

Strain the stock in a large colander set over a large bowl; discard the solids. If desired, strain the stock again through a finer sieve.

Let the stock cool to room temperature, then refrigerate overnight. Skim off and discard the fat on the surface, then transfer the stock to smaller containers.

Makes about 2 quarts

Note: *If you want to use some of the chicken meat for soup or a chicken salad, remove the breasts and/or thighs after 1½ hours and separate the meat from the bones. Then return the bones to the pot and continue simmering. You can also remove a few of the carrots when just tender to reserve for a soup.*

Utilize the space. A full freezer freezes better and uses less energy than an empty one, but you don't want to be pulling out dozens of little packages just to find the chicken breasts you froze 3 months ago. To conserve freezer space, store food in plastic freezer bags rather than in plastic containers. First wrap the food very tightly in foil or plastic wrap, then place the food in a bag, filling it to within ½ inch of the top. Press out as much of the air from the bag as you can and seal. Finally, to make sure you'll know what you've got and how long it's been in the freezer, label the bags with the contents and the date.

Chop and freeze ahead. When prepping for one meal, think about future meals as well. Cut-up vegetables lend themselves to freezing. When you're chopping vegetables for one recipe, simply chop extra and spread out the pieces on a tray to freeze, then divide the frozen pieces into ½-cup portions and store in freezer bags as described above, to use as needed. This works for onions, carrots, bell peppers, celery, leeks, broccoli, spinach, tomatoes, and cauliflower. Fruits freeze well too. Purchase in-season berries, peaches, plums, and nectarines, and freeze as you would chopped vegetables. There's no need to thaw most chopped vegetables or fruits before using.

Cook and freeze ahead. Weekends are a good time to prepare and freeze some dishes for future meals. Soups, stews, chilis, and casseroles all lend themselves to advance cooking. Some baked goods, like the Lemon-Raspberry Muffins on page 32, also freeze well, as do the Multigrain Toaster Waffles on page 251. On days when you know you're going to be pressed from the moment you wake up, you can grab a frozen muffin for a microwave breakfast and pull a stew from the freezer to defrost for a dinner later.

Know when to toss. Most foods will keep up to 6 months in the freezer (although fish and shellfish are best frozen for just a couple of weeks). You can tell if food has been frozen too long if the color has changed dramatically or if it looks dry. Frost on food (or freezer burn) indicates that the food was frozen too slowly or that it has partially thawed and refrozen. If that's the case, get rid of it.

THE SUPERQUICK COOK

Now that you're well versed in shopping and stocking, it's time to get down to the fun part: cooking! The fact that you own this book indicates that while you must love to cook, you're also time challenged. But that doesn't mean you can't get a great meal on the table for yourself, your family, and/or your friends in half an hour or so.

We've said it before and we'll say it again: It all comes down to planning . . . and of course some great gadgets and a few time-saving tricks. Quick cooks know that reading a recipe carefully before you begin can save precious minutes later, as can laying out all your utensils and key ingredients. Professional chefs call this organization *mise en place,* or having the right things in the right place, and it's critical to efficient home cooking, too.

Get the Right Gear

Whether you're slicing, dicing, whipping, or processing, having the right equipment can save on preparation time. Good tools also play a part in helping you maintain your diet and your health. If you've been on the South Beach Diet for a while, you already know that cooking with nonstick skillets, saucepans, and griddles is essential if you want to use less fat. You probably also own a bamboo steamer or collapsible metal steamer for healthy vegetable, chicken, and fish preparation, not to mention a Microplane zester (the best gadget ever) and an instant-read thermometer—all tools we've recommended in previous cookbooks. Today there are more time-saving kitchen appliances and utensils available than ever before. Here are some of our all-time favorites:

Sharp knives. Good sharp knives can really speed up food prep. And you don't have to spend a fortune buying a matching 12-piece set, since all you really need are four: a 3- or 4-inch paring knife for peeling, mincing, and slicing small items; an 8- or 10-inch chef's knife for chopping, dicing, mincing, and julienning, and for slicing meat, fish, and poultry; an 8- or 10-inch carving knife with a slender blade; and a serrated bread knife (which you can also use for slicing tomatoes).

A good knife can be made of carbon steel, stainless steel, or high-carbon stainless; but most people prefer one made from high-carbon stainless because it holds its edge and shiny appearance longer and is easy to sharpen. Handle a knife before buying: It should be solid and well balanced and feel comfortable in your hand.

For maximum sharpness, always keep your knives in a free-standing rack or on a mounted magnetic knife block. Never store them in a kitchen drawer where their delicate edges will be abraded by other gadgets. You don't need to sharpen a knife before each use if you use a sharpening steel to hone the blade to give it a better edge. When honing no longer works and you do need to sharpen, use a whetstone or take your knives to a professional. To clean your knives, always wash by hand, never in the dishwasher. Too much water and harsh detergents can dull and distort both handles and blades.

Kitchen scissors. If you're always using your household shears for kitchen tasks, now is the time to buy a dedicated pair. You'll find endless uses for them, from trimming the excess fat from poultry and beef to snipping out the tough stems from kale.

Y-shaped peeler. With so many fancy peelers on the market, this old-fashioned gadget (with just one moving part) often gets overlooked. Because it easily follows the shape of any fruit or vegetable, it's the fastest way to peel apples and sweet potatoes, make zucchini ribbons, and shave cheese. Look for one with a comfortable handle.

Meat pounder. A number of recipes in this book call for flattening chicken or turkey breasts or pork loin for quicker, more even cooking. Using a meat mallet makes this task a lot easier than banging the poultry with the back of a heavy skillet.

Immersion blender (aka stick blender). This handheld tool makes easy work of puréeing soups, sauces, dips, and smoothies. It has a long, narrow stem with rotary blades at the end so you can blend or purée foods right in the pot, bowl, or glass and avoid dirtying the food processor or blender. Look for one with a powerful motor that is lightweight enough to hold comfortably. Cordless models offer the greatest convenience.

Mini food processor. This indispensable gadget is available with a bowl capacity of 1½ to 3 cups. It doesn't take up much space on your counter and comes in handy for speedily chopping herbs, garlic, and nuts. It's also great for grinding flaxseed for flaxmeal (see page 147 for how we use flaxmeal in a cheeseburger), making whole-wheat bread crumbs, and grating cheese. Make sure the one you buy has a good-size feed tube.

Slow cooker. Sometimes quicker cooking means slower cooking. With a slow cooker you can get a dinner going early in the day and forget about it until it's time to eat. Or, in a reverse move, you can use the slow cooker overnight to make a healthy breakfast. On page 250 we include a recipe for steel-cut oatmeal that can be started when you go to bed and enjoyed in the morning (and it's good for days afterward). Slow cookers are also a boon for making large-batch soups, chilis, and stews to freeze for later use.

Maximize Your Kitchen Time

As we created the dishes for this book, we did so with an eye toward your busy lifestyle, noting cooking times on each. We also realize that you may not necessarily be cooking for a family of four. If that's the case, remember that you can easily cut many of the recipes in this book in half to serve two (or one, with leftovers for another day). See the box, opposite, for some suggestions on which recipes will adapt to smaller servings most readily. Those recipes that offer "Cook Once, Eat Twice" suggestions are also well suited to cooking for fewer than four, as you can serve half one night and transform the leftovers for another meal later on with no need to double the original recipe. And for those days when you don't even want to turn the stove or oven on, look to no-cook recipes like Confetti Crab Salad (page 87), Curried Turkey Salad (page 89), and Quick Cobb Salad (page 93) or one of the other simple no-cook salads we suggest on page 18. Lastly, many of our recipes are perfect grab-and-go solutions; see the list of breakfasts, lunches, and snacks on the following pages.

About Our Grab-and-Go Dishes

While we don't recommend eating on the run too often, there will always be those hectic times when you'll need to take along food rather than skip a meal or snack. The following are some recipes from the book that lend themselves to grab-and-go breakfasts, lunches, and snacks, plus some additional ideas for take-away breakfast burritos, smoothies, superquick soups, and more.

For mess-free transport, invest in some small plastic containers and cups in several sizes (ideally, some should be microwave safe) and make sure they have tight-fitting lids. Plastic wrap works well for the muffins, burgers, and wraps.

Quick Dishes for Two

Many of the recipes in this book can easily be halved to make delicious meals for two people. Just remember to use a smaller skillet and/or baking sheet to accommodate the smaller number of servings. Here are a few dishes that lend themselves especially well to being halved:

Fruit and Yogurt Breakfast Parfaits (page 25, Phase 2)

Ham and Cheese Frico Breakwiches (page 30, Phase 1)

Individual Pizzas with Gruyère, Caramelized Onions, and Apples (page 187, Phase 2)

Baby Greens and Grilled Asparagus with Shallot Vinaigrette (page 224, Phase 1)

Indian-Spiced Mashed Sweet Potatoes (page 218, Phase 2)

Roasted Green and Wax Beans with Walnuts (page 211, Phase 1)

Shrimp Fra Diavolo (page 124, Phase 1)

Garlic Shrimp with Swiss Chard and Chickpeas (page 117, Phase 1)

Roasted Pecan Salmon with Lentil-Tomato Salad (page 108, Phase 1)

Sole à la Meunière (page 112, Phase 1)

Tilapia Margarita (page 114, Phase 1)

Baked Halibut with Asparagus and Shiitake Mushrooms (page 122, Phase 1)

Striped Bass Roasted with Cauliflower, Lemon, and Olives (page 109, Phase 1)

Peppered Chicken Cutlets (page 149, Phase 1)

Crispy Chicken Fingers (page 144, Phase 2)

Lemon-Caper Chicken (page 155, Phase 2)

Chicken with Spicy Roasted Tomato-Leek Sauce (page 161, Phase 1)

Spicy Pork Skewers with Cashew Sauce (page 167, Phase 1)

Texas Bowl o' Red (page 182, Phase 1)

Grilled Summer Fruits (page 244, Phase 2)

Glazed Bananas with Lime Cream (page 234, Phase 2)

Mini Breakfast Frittata (page 28, Phase 1): Wrap a frittata in plastic wrap for easy travel or put in a whole-wheat pita or tortilla if you're on Phase 2.

Overnight Oatmeal (page 250, Phase 2): Pack a portion of oatmeal in a microwavable container and take it to the office to reheat for an easy breakfast (or even lunch).

Lemon-Raspberry Muffins (page 32, Phase 2): Make a big batch of muffins, wrap them individually, and then freeze for up to 3 months. Take along to work and enjoy with yogurt for breakfast or a snack.

Fruit and Yogurt Breakfast Parfait (page 25, Phase 2): Layer the ingredients into a 8-ounce travel cup with lid or a disposable paper coffee cup with a lid.

Apricot-Oat Bars (page 36, Phase 2): Wrap the bars individually and pop them into the freezer, where they will keep for 3 months. Pack one in your purse or backpack and it will be thawed by the time you're ready to enjoy it.

Broccoli, Pepper, and Cheese Bites (page 41, Phase 1): Take a couple of these along for breakfast, lunch, or a snack. They're delicious at room temperature or microwaved. If you're on Phase 2, they make a great sandwich with whole-grain bread.

Tofu, Spinach, and Egg Scramble (page 29, Phase 1): If you're on Phase 2, wrap in a tortilla and plastic wrap for a take-away morning meal.

Peanut Butter Cheese Crackers (Phase 2): Spread a few whole-wheat crackers with a little natural no-sugar-added peanut butter and top with a piece of reduced-fat Cheddar cheese and another cracker. Wrap well in plastic wrap.

Blueberry-Mango Smoothie (Phase 2): Toss ½ cup fresh or frozen blueberries into a blender along with 1 cup reduced-fat soy milk, ½ cup cubed mango, and 1 tablespoon flaxmeal. Purée until smooth. The smoothie can be poured into a cup and frozen or taken along as is.

Banana-Sunflower Smoothie (Phase 2): In a blender, combine a banana, ¾ cup fat-free milk, 2 tablespoons sunflower butter, 1 tablespoon nonfat dry milk powder, and 1 tablespoon sugar-free chocolate syrup; purée until smooth. Pour into ice cube trays and freeze, then pop out 4 (for a ½-cup serving), and transfer to a lidded cup for carrying. It will be ready to drink when you arrive.

Tofu–Mixed Berry Smoothie (Phase 2): In a blender, combine 8 ounces soft silken tofu, 1 cup frozen mixed berries (no need to thaw), a little granular sugar substitute, and a little pure vanilla extract. Purée until thick and smooth. The smoothie can be poured into a lidded cup and taken along.

Breakfast Bean Burrito (Phase 2): Mash canned or cooked black beans with a little chopped garlic, extra-virgin olive oil, and chopped scallion; season with chili powder and a squeeze of fresh lime juice. Spread on a whole-wheat tortilla. Add thin strips of red and green bell pepper and roll up. Wrap in foil for carrying.

Breakfast Egg and Cheese Burrito (Phase 2): Beat a couple of eggs and slowly cook in a small nonstick skillet. Just before the eggs are done, add reduced-fat shredded Cheddar cheese, thinly sliced scallion, and a little paprika. Cook until the cheese has melted. Pile onto a whole-wheat tortilla and roll up. Wrap in foil for carrying.

Yogurt, Cottage Cheese, Fruit, and Nut Combo (Phase 2): Combine equal amounts of low-fat cottage cheese and nonfat Greek yogurt. Add some blueberries, some sliced natural almonds, and a little agave nectar or granular sugar substitute; stir well. Carry in a lidded cup.

Herbed Greek Yogurt (Phase 1): Stir together nonfat Greek yogurt, chopped chives and parsley, and black pepper. Carry in a lidded cup.

Grab-and-Go Lunches

Shrimp Cone (page 71, Phase 2): Roll up like a burrito, then wrap tightly in plastic wrap for carrying. Refrigerate if not eating immediately.

Asian Beef in Lettuce Cups (page 77, Phase 1): Pack the beef mixture and lettuce separately in plastic containers and assemble when ready to eat, or omit the lettuce and just have the beef mixture as a salad.

Asian Roast Pork Salad (page 102, Phase 2): Combine all the salad ingredients, except the Asian pear. Thinly slice the pear and toss with a little lemon juice and wrap separately. Refrigerate both until ready to eat, then combine.

Buffalo Chicken Salad (page 104, Phase 1): Omit the greens, toss the remaining ingredients together, and pack in an airtight container. Refrigerate until ready to eat.

Inside-Out Cheeseburger (page 147, Phase 2): Wrap a chilled burger in

10 Simple No-Cook Salads

1. **Arugula, Sun-Dried Tomato, and Ricotta Salata Salad** (Phase 1): Toss arugula, chopped sun-dried tomatoes, romaine lettuce, black olives, ricotta salata, chopped celery and celery leaves, and sliced mushrooms with a mustard vinaigrette.

2. **Shrimp, Radicchio, and Fennel Salad** (Phase 1): Toss cooked shrimp with torn pieces of radicchio, shaved fennel, fresh lemon juice, extra-virgin olive oil, and grated Parmesan.

3. **Tuna-Chickpea Salad** (Phase 1): Toss drained water-packed tuna with chickpeas, diced red bell pepper, sliced red onion, shredded basil, and extra-virgin olive oil.

4. **Artichoke Salad** (Phase 1): Combine rinsed and drained water-packed artichoke hearts, coarsely chopped hard-boiled eggs, and chopped plum tomatoes. Toss with a little mayo and red wine vinegar.

5. **Quick Chicken Salad** (Phase 1): Make a dressing of chopped anchovies or anchovy paste, a little mayo, fresh lemon juice, and a pinch of cayenne. Add pieces of grilled, roasted, or rotisserie skinless chicken breast, slices of cucumber, and sliced hearts of palm.

plastic wrap or a whole-wheat pita. Enjoy at room temperature or briefly reheat in a microwave oven.

Seven-Vegetable Salad (page 82, Phase 2): Pack in a travel container and eat chilled or at room temperature.

Italian Tuna Burger (page 133, Phase 2): Pack in a whole-wheat pita and wrap in plastic wrap.

Mini Turkey Meatloaf (page 141, Phase 2): This is delicious warm (reheat in the microwave) or at room temperature. Enjoy with a salad on the side. Wrap in plastic wrap for carrying.

Satay Chicken Burger (page 152, Phase 1): The burger can be eaten chilled

6. **Greek Feta Salad** (Phase 1): Toss shredded romaine lettuce with thinly sliced scallions, chopped dill, crumbled reduced-fat feta cheese, fresh lemon juice, extra-virgin olive oil, salt, and pepper.

7. **Spicy Beef Salad** (Phase 1): Combine a few tablespoons of light sour cream with a few tablespoons of mayonnaise. Add chipotle chile powder to taste, along with chopped pickles, sliced cucumbers, pepperoncini, and thin strips of deli roast beef. Serve on a bed of romaine or mesclun.

8. **Turkey Reuben Salad** (Phase 1): Rinse and drain sauerkraut and toss with shredded red cabbage, thin strips of reduced-fat Swiss cheese, thin strips of deli turkey breast, and a light dressing of mayo and tomato paste.

9. **Thai Beef Salad** (Phase 2): Make a dressing of fish sauce or soy sauce, dark sesame oil, extra-virgin olive oil, and fresh lemon juice. Toss with shredded cabbage and carrot, thinly sliced red bell pepper, and lean deli roast beef.

10. **Tropical Black Bean Salad** (Phase 2): Toss rinsed and drained canned black beans with a spicy hot sauce, diced papaya, halved cherry or grape tomatoes, sliced scallions, fresh lime juice, extra-virgin olive oil, and chunks of reduced-fat Monterey Jack cheese.

or at room temperature. Wrap in plastic wrap for carrying. Pack a little Chinese Peanut Sauce (page 228) separately to drizzle on top.

Mushroom-Beef Burger with Watercress Cream (page 178, Phase 2): The burger is great at room temp. Wrap it in plastic wrap for carrying, with the horseradish cream (for spreading or dipping) packed separately.

Eggplant Caprese (page 186, Phase 1): Pack in a plastic container and enjoy chilled or microwaved. If you're on Phase 2, enjoy in a wrap.

Asparagus and Red Pepper Frittata with Goat Cheese (page 193, Phase 1): Pack a wedge of frittata along with a side salad and some low-sugar prepared dressing of your choice (packed separately).

Crispy Chicken Fingers (page 144, Phase 2): These are good at room temperature or chilled. Bring along some Mango Salsa (page 227) or Dijon mustard for dipping, or a wedge of lemon for squeezing.

Pesto Pasta Salad (page 92, Phase 2): This is delicious served at room temperature or chilled.

Double-Soy Salad (page 99, Phase 1): Omit the romaine lettuce, pack the salad in a travel container, then refrigerate until ready to eat.

Smoked Turkey Roll-Ups with Lemony Avocado Spread (page 68, Phase 1): Wrap the roll-up tightly in plastic wrap for carrying.

Quick Minestrone Soup (Phase 1): Make this 10-minute soup first thing in the morning: Heat vegetable broth, then add a little tomato paste, some cut-up green beans, sliced yellow squash and zucchini, and some canned white beans. Pour into a wide-mouth thermos. Carry along some grated Parmesan cheese.

Asian Chicken Vegetable Soup (Phase 1): Here's another fast-to-prepare take-along soup: Heat lower-sodium chicken broth. Add grated ginger, chunks of firm tofu, some shredded cabbage, a little dark sesame oil, and a splash of rice vinegar. Pour into a wide-mouth thermos.

Turkey-Cheddar Roll (Phase 1): Spread 2 thin slices of deli turkey breast with a little Dijon mustard and wrap around strips of reduced-fat Cheddar. For Phase 2, add some pear slices. Wrap tightly in plastic wrap.

Grab-and-Go Snacks

Smoked-Trout Deviled Eggs (page 51, Phase 1): Wrap the stuffed eggs individually in plastic wrap to take with you, then refrigerate until ready to eat.

Shrimp Cocktail with Creamy Chipotle Sauce (page 45, Phase 1): Pack individual portions of the shrimp and sauce in plastic containers. Refrigerate if you're not eating immediately.

Roasted Adobo Lentils (page 54, Phase 1): The lentils will keep in an airtight container at room temperature for up to a week. Pack a little bag of them for the road.

South Beach Diet Snack Mix (page 55, Phase 2): Pack in a small resealable plastic bag or reusable container and carry along for midmorning munching.

Spinach and Artichoke Dip (page 49, Phase 1): This dip is great with

Postworkout Snacking

Whatever phase of the diet you're on, exercise is essential for achieving and maintaining your weight loss. Snacking after exercise allows you to recover lost energy and prepare for the next activity in your day. Research suggests that the best postworkout snack is a combination of protein and good carbohydrates.

The amount you eat will depend on the length and intensity of your workout. If you're doing 20 minutes of interval or core training, for example (which Dr. Agatston describes in his book *The South Beach Diet Supercharged*), then you probably won't need to refuel. But for those who participate in sustained high-intensity workouts, a snack can be essential.

If you're on Phase 1, have fat-free or low-fat plain yogurt, natural peanut butter, a 2-ounce container of hummus, a little reduced-fat cheese, or a slice or two of a lean deli meat with some veggies. Or enjoy our Double-Nut Snack (below). On Phase 2 you can have the same, plus a slice of whole-wheat bread or a whole-wheat pita. Our South Beach Diet Snack Mix (page 55) is also good for Phase 2 exercisers.

Remember to snack within 15 minutes after your workout—glycogen fuel stores are more rapidly replaced during this short window of time. Also be sure to drink plenty of water to replenish the fluids you lose when sweating.

crudités. If you're on Phase 2, it makes a good spread for whole-wheat crackers. Pack dip and dippers in separate containers.

Red Pepper, Feta, and Mint Dip (page 50, Phase 1): Carry the dip along with some crunchy vegetables—or a whole-wheat pita if you're on Phase 2.

Whole-Wheat Avocado Bread (page 252, Phase 2): Cut and freeze individual slices in plastic wrap and then put the frozen slices in a larger freezer container. Grab a slice in its wrapper to eat as a midmorning snack; it thaws quickly.

Double-Nut Snack (Phase 1): Combine soy nuts, toasted almonds, and crumbled sheets of nori for a quick high-protein snack.

Spicy Hard-Boiled Eggs (Phase 1): Pack 2 hard-boiled egg halves to eat with a separate sauce of puréed cilantro, parsley, jalapeño pepper, garlic, and a little extra-virgin olive oil.

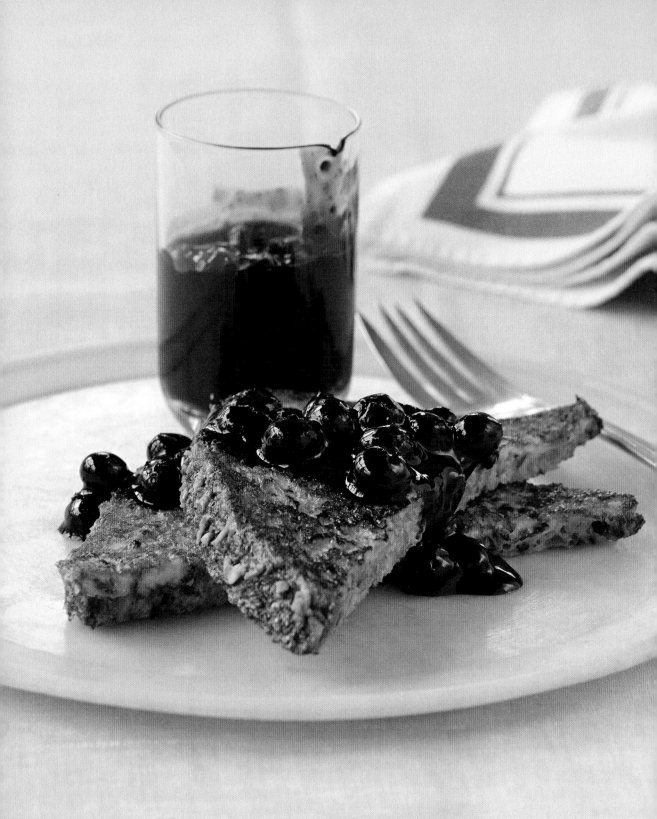

Almond French Toast with Warm Blueberry Syrup (page 24)

BREAKFASTS

We all know how important it is to start the day with a healthy breakfast—a remarkable 92 percent of Americans consider it *the* most important meal of the day. Yet only 46 percent of us eat breakfast of any kind 7 days a week, allowing crazy morning schedules to turn breakfast into an afterthought.

On the South Beach Diet we don't want you to skip breakfast no matter how busy you are. Studies show that a high-protein meal for breakfast (such as eggs and Canadian bacon) provides a greater sense of fullness than when the same amount of protein is eaten at lunch or dinner. Moreover, people who regularly eat two eggs for breakfast as part of a reduced-calorie diet lose more weight and feel more energetic than those who eat bagel breakfasts of equal calories.

In this chapter we offer ideas for sit-down morning meals you can prepare in half an hour or less, as well as easy-to-transport breakfasts to eat on the road or at the office.

Almond French Toast with Warm Blueberry Syrup

MAKES 4 servings   **HANDS-ON TIME: 15 minutes**   **TOTAL TIME: 20 minutes**

If you have a large enough skillet to hold all the bread in one layer, make the French toast in just one batch. You can make extra syrup to have on hand for breakfasts later on; it will keep in the fridge for up to a week.

BLUEBERRY SYRUP

- 2 cups frozen unsweetened blueberries
- 2 teaspoons fresh lime juice
- 2 teaspoons granular sugar substitute, or to taste

FRENCH TOAST

- 2 large eggs
- ½ cup fat-free or 1% milk
- 1 tablespoon granular sugar substitute
- ½ teaspoon pure almond extract
- ¼ teaspoon salt

  Pinch grated nutmeg
- 4 slices whole-grain bread
- 4 teaspoons light olive oil

For the syrup: In a nonaluminum saucepan, bring the blueberries to a simmer over medium heat and cook until the berries burst and the sauce thickens, about 12 minutes. Remove the pan from the heat and stir in the lime juice. Stir in the sugar substitute; taste for sweetness and add more sugar substitute, if desired. Keep warm.

While the berries are cooking, make the French toast: In a shallow bowl, whisk together the eggs, milk, sugar substitute, almond extract, salt, and nutmeg. Add 2 slices of the bread and soak for 30 seconds per side. Repeat with the remaining slices.

In a nonstick skillet, heat 2 teaspoons of the oil over medium heat, swirling to coat the bottom of the pan. Add 2 bread slices and cook until golden brown, about 1½ minutes per side. Transfer to a plate and keep warm. Repeat with the remaining 2 teaspoons oil and bread.

Serve the French toast with ¼ cup warm blueberry syrup per serving.

NUTRITION AT A GLANCE
Per serving with ¼ cup syrup: 173 calories, 8 g fat, 4.5 g saturated fat, 6 g protein, 21 g carbohydrate, 6 g fiber, 277 mg sodium

Fruit and Yogurt Breakfast Parfaits

MAKES 4 (1-cup) servings   **HANDS-ON TIME: 10 minutes**   **TOTAL TIME: 10 minutes**

15 MINUTE RECIPE

Adding nonfat dry milk to Greek yogurt rounds out the flavor, making it a little less tart. It also adds additional protein and calcium to the parfaits. Covered tightly with plastic wrap, the parfaits hold up beautifully in the fridge.

- 2 small ripe bananas, cut up
- 2 small nectarines, cubed
- 1 teaspoon plus 2 tablespoons granular sugar substitute
- 1 teaspoon pure vanilla extract
- 2 cups nonfat (0%) plain Greek yogurt
- ¼ cup nonfat dry milk powder

In a food processor or blender, purée the bananas, nectarines, 1 teaspoon of the sugar substitute, and ½ teaspoon of the vanilla.

In a medium bowl, whisk together the yogurt and milk powder. Whisk in the remaining 2 tablespoons sugar substitute and ½ teaspoon vanilla.

Spoon ½ cup of the banana-nectarine mixture into each of four 8-ounce glasses. Top each with ½ cup of the yogurt mixture. Serve right away or cover and refrigerate for up to 3 days.

NUTRITION AT A GLANCE
Per serving: 155 calories, 0.4 g fat, 0 g saturated fat, 13 g protein, 26 g carbohydrate, 2 g fiber, 68 mg sodium

TIP: These parfaits travel well in plastic cups and make a great on-the-go breakfast or snack.

Poached Eggs Arrabbiata

MAKES 4 servings   HANDS-ON TIME: 10 minutes   TOTAL TIME: 30 minutes

These easy eggs, which poach in a rich red sauce, are perfect for a relaxed brunch. Red pepper flakes add a touch of heat; add more or less to your taste, or pass at the table. The addition of feta provides extra protein.

2 teaspoons extra-virgin olive oil

1 small green bell pepper, cut into ½-inch dice

1 small onion, finely chopped

1 garlic clove, thinly sliced

1 can (15 ounces) crushed tomatoes

¼ teaspoon red pepper flakes

¼ teaspoon salt

4 large eggs

½ cup reduced-fat feta cheese, crumbled (2 ounces)

Cracked black pepper

In a large nonstick skillet, heat the oil over medium heat. Add the bell pepper, onion, garlic, and 2 tablespoons water. Cook, stirring frequently, until the vegetables are tender, about 7 minutes. Add the tomatoes and their liquid, pepper flakes, and salt. Bring to a boil, then reduce to a simmer.

Working with 1 egg at a time, carefully crack an egg into a cup. With the lip of the cup at the inside edge of the pan, slip the egg into the simmering sauce. When all the eggs have been added, cover the skillet and cook for about 2 minutes.

Uncover the pan, spoon some sauce over the eggs, and continue to cook, covered, for another 10 minutes, or until the eggs are set.

Spoon 1 egg and some sauce into each of 4 bowls. Sprinkle each serving with 2 tablespoons of the feta and some black pepper and serve.

NUTRITION AT A GLANCE
Per serving: 168 calories, 10 g fat, 3 g saturated fat, 11 g protein, 11 g carbohydrate, 3 g fiber, 553 mg sodium

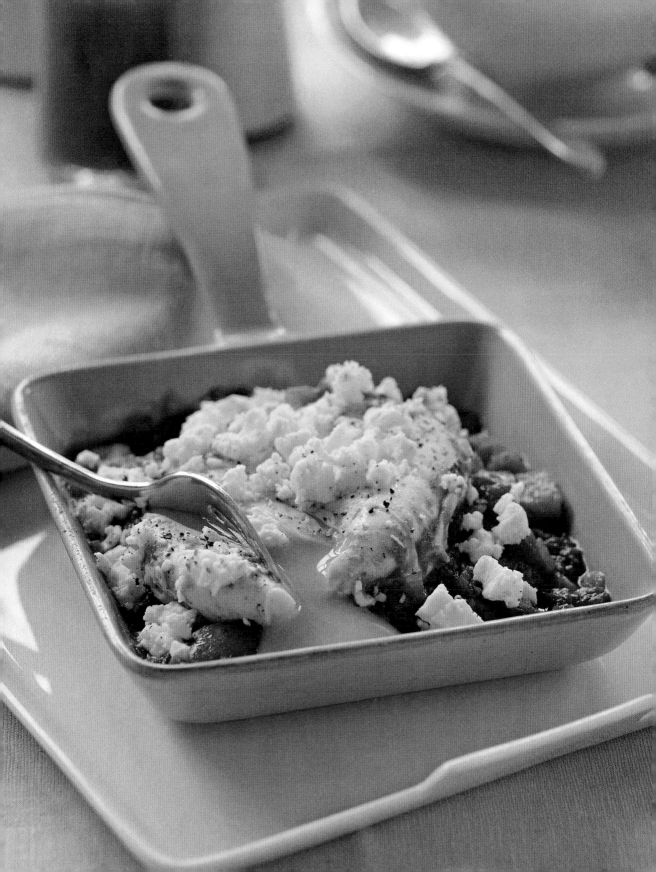

Mini Breakfast Frittatas

MAKES 12 mini frittatas (3 per serving)   HANDS-ON TIME: 10 minutes   TOTAL TIME: 30 minutes

If you love a morning omelet, here's one you can take on the road. A variation on our popular Vegetable Quiche Cups to Go recipe, these little omelets are great right out of the oven but can also be served at room temperature. Store the well-wrapped frittatas in the refrigerator for up to a week.

- 1 package (10 ounces) frozen cut green beans
- 4 sun-dried tomato halves (in oil)
- 2 scallions, cut into 1-inch pieces
- 1 teaspoon Italian herb blend
- ¼ teaspoon salt
- 1¼ cups egg substitute
- ¾ cup shredded part-skim mozzarella cheese (3 ounces)
- Black pepper

Heat the oven to 350°F. Coat a 12-cup muffin pan with cooking spray, or use a nonstick pan.

Place the green beans in a strainer and run hot water over them to thaw. Drain well, pressing to get out as much liquid as possible.

Combine the beans, sun-dried tomatoes, scallions, herb blend, and salt in a food processor. Pulse on and off to chop coarsely. Add the egg substitute and pulse just to combine.

Spoon 2 tablespoons of the mixture into each muffin cup. Top each with 1 tablespoon cheese. Season the tops with a grind of pepper. Bake for 20 minutes, or until a toothpick inserted in the center comes out clean. Serve warm or at room temperature.

NUTRITION AT A GLANCE
Per frittata: 44 calories, 2 g fat, 1 g saturated fat, 5 g protein, 3 g carbohydrate, 1 g fiber, 152 mg sodium

Tofu, Spinach, and Egg Scramble

MAKES 4 servings   HANDS-ON TIME: 15 minutes   TOTAL TIME: 20 minutes

Frozen chopped spinach—a great item to keep on hand—is perfect for a quick-cooking breakfast. Just remember to squeeze it dry once it's been thawed so the scramble isn't watery.

4 teaspoons extra-virgin olive oil

6 ounces lite firm tofu, patted dry and cut into 1-inch chunks

1 package (10 ounces) frozen chopped spinach, thawed and squeezed dry

¼ cup chopped fresh dill or basil

¾ teaspoon salt

3 large eggs

2 large egg whites (¼ cup)

½ avocado, cut into ½-inch dice

In a large nonstick skillet, heat 2 teaspoons of the oil over medium heat. Add the tofu and cook, tossing occasionally, until golden brown, about 5 minutes. With a slotted spoon, transfer to a plate and keep warm.

Add the remaining 2 teaspoons oil, the spinach, dill, and ¼ teaspoon of the salt to the skillet and cook, stirring occasionally, until the spinach is tender, about 3 minutes.

Meanwhile, in a large bowl, whisk together the eggs, egg whites, remaining ½ teaspoon salt, and 2 tablespoons water.

Add the egg mixture to pan with the spinach and cook, stirring, until eggs are almost set, about 1 minute. Gently fold in the tofu. Divide evenly among 4 plates and top with the avocado.

NUTRITION AT A GLANCE
Per serving: 177 calories, 12 g fat, 2 g saturated fat, 13 g protein, 6 g carbohydrate, 4 g fiber, 584 mg sodium

15 MINUTE RECIPE

Ham and Cheese Frico Breakwiches

MAKES 4 sandwiches   **HANDS-ON TIME:** 10 minutes   **TOTAL TIME:** 15 minutes

This unusual, quick-to-make breakfast sandwich uses homemade *frico,* or cheese crisps, instead of bread. If you prefer, you can fill the sandwiches with smoked turkey or Canadian bacon instead of ham and use shredded Parmesan instead of sharp Cheddar to make the cheese crisps.

- 1 cup shredded reduced-fat sharp Cheddar cheese (4 ounces)
- 4 teaspoons coarse-grain mustard
- 2 ounces sliced smoked ham, cut into 8 pieces
- 4 roasted red pepper halves (from a jar)
- ¼ cup thinly sliced red onion

Heat the oven to 375°F. Line a baking sheet with parchment paper.

Using 2 tablespoons for each, sprinkle the cheese into 8 mounds on the baking sheet. Spread each mound out into a 3-inch round. Bake for 3 minutes, or until the cheese has melted and spread slightly. Remove from the oven and let stand on the baking sheet until the cheese sets, about 2 minutes.

Using a thin-bladed metal spatula, lift the rounds off the baking sheet. Brush the smooth side of each round with mustard. Top each of 4 rounds with 1 piece of ham, a red pepper, another piece of ham, and one-fourth of the onion. Top with the remaining cheese rounds, mustard side down, and serve warm.

NUTRITION AT A GLANCE
Per sandwich: 123 calories, 6 g fat, 4 g saturated fat, 10 g protein, 6 g carbohydrate, 1 g fiber, 495 mg sodium

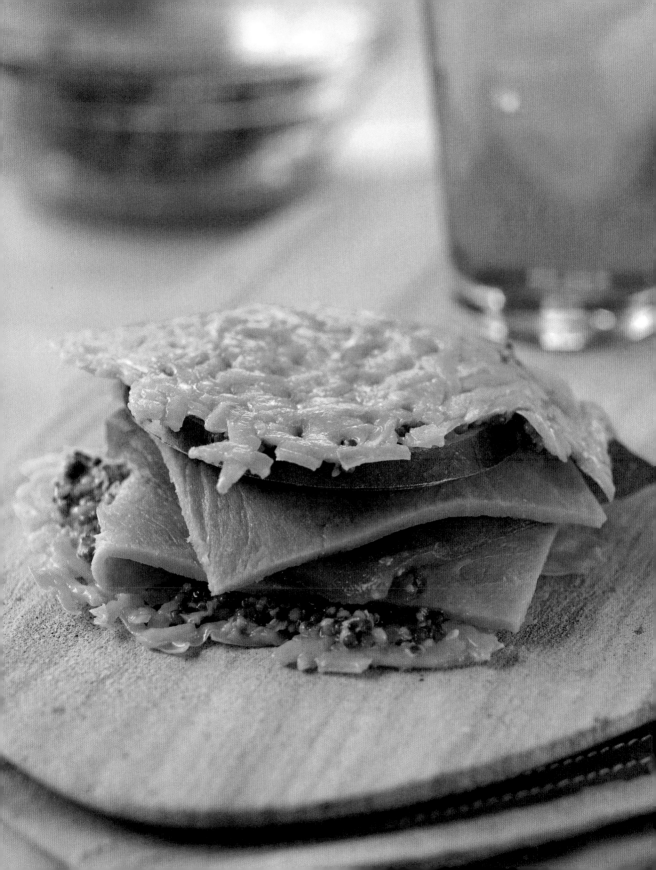

Lemon-Raspberry Muffins

MAKES 12 muffins (1 per serving)   HANDS-ON TIME: 10 minutes   TOTAL TIME: 30 minutes

Enjoy one of these healthy muffins for breakfast with a glass of low-fat or fat-free milk for protein (the quinoa flakes provide additional complete protein). Look for quinoa flakes (a great substitute for oats in baked goods) with the grains in health-food stores. If you prefer a sweeter muffin, add a little more granular sugar substitute to your taste.

1 cup quinoa flakes

1 cup whole-wheat flour

2 tablespoons granular sugar substitute

2 teaspoons baking powder

1 teaspoon grated lemon zest

½ teaspoon baking soda

¼ teaspoon salt

¾ cup light (1.5%) buttermilk

3 tablespoons safflower oil or canola oil

1 large egg

1 cup fresh raspberries, or 1 cup frozen raspberries, thawed and drained

Heat the oven to 375°F. Line a 12-cup muffin tin with paper liners.

In a large bowl, stir together the quinoa flakes, flour, sugar substitute, baking powder, lemon zest, baking soda, and salt.

In another large bowl, whisk together the buttermilk, oil, and egg. Make a well in the center of the dry ingredients, add the buttermilk mixture, and fold until just combined. Fold in the raspberries.

Spoon the batter into the muffin cups and bake for 20 minutes, or until a toothpick inserted in the center of a muffin comes out clean.

NUTRITION AT A GLANCE

Per muffin: 109 calories, 4.5 g fat, 0.5 g saturated fat, 3 g protein, 15 g carbohydrate, 2 g fiber, 240 mg sodium

TIP: Use an ice cream scoop to portion out the muffin batter quickly and evenly.

South Beach Diet Breakfast Bowl

MAKES 4 servings   HANDS-ON TIME: 15 minutes   TOTAL TIME: 15 minutes

Seems like the breakfast bowl concept has taken over many fast-food chains—but who says a breakfast bowl has to include white potatoes, pork sausage, and full-fat cheese? This healthy version uses both whole eggs and egg whites, replaces the typical fried potatoes with fiber-rich beans, and uses healthy monounsaturated avocado instead of the cheese. Be sure to choose a jarred salsa that has no sugar added.

1 can (15.5 ounces) pinto beans, rinsed and drained

1 cup no-sugar-added prepared salsa

4 large eggs

3 large egg whites (6 tablespoons)

½ teaspoon ground cumin

¼ teaspoon black pepper

2 teaspoons extra-virgin olive oil

1 teaspoon trans-fat-free margarine (vegetable oil spread)

1 avocado, thinly sliced

In a small saucepan, combine the beans and ½ cup of the salsa. Warm over very low heat while you cook the eggs.

In a medium bowl, whisk together the whole eggs, egg whites, cumin, and pepper. In a medium nonstick skillet, heat the oil and margarine over medium heat. Add the egg mixture and cook, without stirring, for 1 minute. Lift the edges and let uncooked egg run underneath. Cook, stirring, until the eggs are set but still moist, 2 to 3 minutes longer.

For each serving, place one-fourth of the beans (scant ½ cup) and one-fourth of the eggs in a shallow soup bowl. Top each portion with 2 tablespoons of the remaining salsa and one-fourth of the avocado.

NUTRITION AT A GLANCE
Per serving: 256 calories, 14 g fat, 3 g saturated fat, 13 g protein, 19 g carbohydrate, 6 g fiber, 688 mg sodium

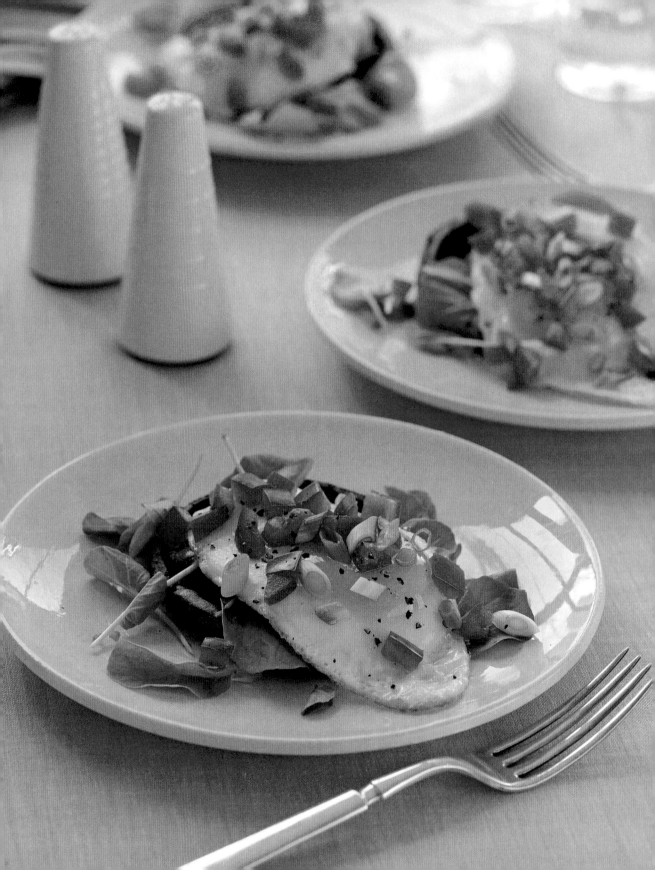

"Fried" Eggs in Mushroom Caps

MAKES 4 servings   HANDS-ON TIME: 10 minutes   TOTAL TIME: 20 minutes

Meaty portobello mushrooms are the healthy base for this egg breakfast: The addition of water to the skillet allows you to "fry" the eggs in just a little oil, with trans-fat-free margarine added for flavor. If you can find one of the vegetable oil spreads with heart-healthy sterols and stanols added, use it.

4   medium portobello mushroom caps (3 ounces each), stems removed

2   teaspoons extra-virgin olive oil

1   tablespoon balsamic vinegar

2   teaspoons trans-fat-free margarine (vegetable oil spread)

4   large eggs

½   teaspoon salt

⅓   cup grated Parmesan cheese

1   cup watercress sprigs, thick stems removed

1   plum tomato, diced

2   scallions, thinly sliced

Freshly ground black pepper (optional)

With a teaspoon, scrape out the gills of each mushroom cap and discard. In a large nonstick skillet, whisk together 1 teaspoon of the oil, the vinegar, and ¼ cup water. Add the mushroom caps, stemmed sides down, and bring to a simmer over medium heat. Reduce the heat, cover, and cook for 5 minutes, or until the mushrooms are tender. Drain and set the mushrooms aside.

In the same skillet, heat the remaining 1 teaspoon oil, the margarine, and 2 tablespoons water over medium heat. When the margarine has melted, crack the eggs into the pan and sprinkle with the salt. Cover and cook for about 5 minutes, until the eggs are set.

Place a mushroom cap, stemmed side up, on each of 4 plates. Divide the Parmesan evenly among the caps and top each with watercress, an egg, and some tomato and scallions. Serve hot, sprinkled with black pepper, if desired.

NUTRITION AT A GLANCE
Per serving: 172 calories, 11 g fat, 3.5 g saturated fat, 11 g protein, 7 g carbohydrate, 2 g fiber, 490 mg sodium

Apricot-Oat Bars

MAKES 12 bars (1 per serving)   HANDS-ON TIME: 10 minutes   TOTAL TIME: 25 minutes

This recipe calls for peanut butter and apricots, but you can substitute another no-sugar-added nut butter (try cashew) and use dried cranberries or chopped dried apples or pears instead of the apricots.

½ cup natural creamy no-sugar-added peanut butter

1 teaspoon pure vanilla extract

2 cups old-fashioned (not instant) rolled oats

⅔ cup dried apricots, coarsely chopped

½ cup walnut halves, coarsely chopped

¼ cup granular sugar substitute

3 large egg whites (6 tablespoons)

¼ teaspoon salt

Heat the oven to 350°F. Line a 9 × 9-inch baking pan with parchment, leaving a 2-inch overhang on 2 sides.

In a large bowl, whisk together the peanut butter, vanilla, and ¼ cup water. Add the oats, apricots, walnuts, sugar substitute, egg whites, and salt. Mix with your hands to combine. Transfer to the pan and pat with moistened hands until even. Bake for 15 minutes, or until crisp and set.

Cool in the pan briefly, then using the overhang, lift out of the pan. Cut immediately into twelve 3 × 2½-inch bars.

NUTRITION AT A GLANCE
Per bar: 154 calories, 9 g fat, 1 g saturated fat, 7 g protein, 12 g carbohydrate, 2 g fiber, 62 mg sodium

Fluffy Berry-Studded Pancakes

MAKES 8 pancakes (2 per serving)   HANDS-ON TIME: 10 minutes   TOTAL TIME: 20 minutes

If there is too much liquid in your cottage cheese, drain it in a strainer before mixing it with the other ingredients. You can use whole raspberries or sliced strawberries instead of blueberries; choose what looks best at the market. Serve the pancakes with sugar-free maple syrup, if desired.

8 ounces low-fat (1%) cottage cheese

¼ cup whole-wheat flour

2 tablespoons granular sugar substitute

½ teaspoon baking powder

¼ teaspoon salt

1 large egg

2 tablespoons plus 2 teaspoons safflower oil or canola oil

1 teaspoon grated orange zest

⅓ cup fresh blueberries, or ⅓ cup frozen blueberries, thawed and drained

In a large bowl, stir together the cottage cheese, flour, sugar substitute, baking powder, and salt. Stir in the egg, 2 tablespoons of the oil, and the orange zest.

In a large nonstick skillet, heat 1 teaspoon of the oil over medium heat. Drop half of the batter into the skillet by rounded tablespoons, making 4 pancakes. Cook until the tops are bubbly and the pancakes are set, about 2 minutes. Scatter half of the blueberries over the tops and press in gently. Turn the pancakes over and cook until firm and set, 1 to 2 minutes longer. Transfer to a plate and keep warm.

Repeat with the remaining 1 teaspoon oil, the batter, and blueberries. Serve warm.

NUTRITION AT A GLANCE

Per pancake: 155 calories, 9 g fat, 1 g saturated fat, 10 g protein, 10 g carbohydrate, 1 g fiber, 444 mg sodium

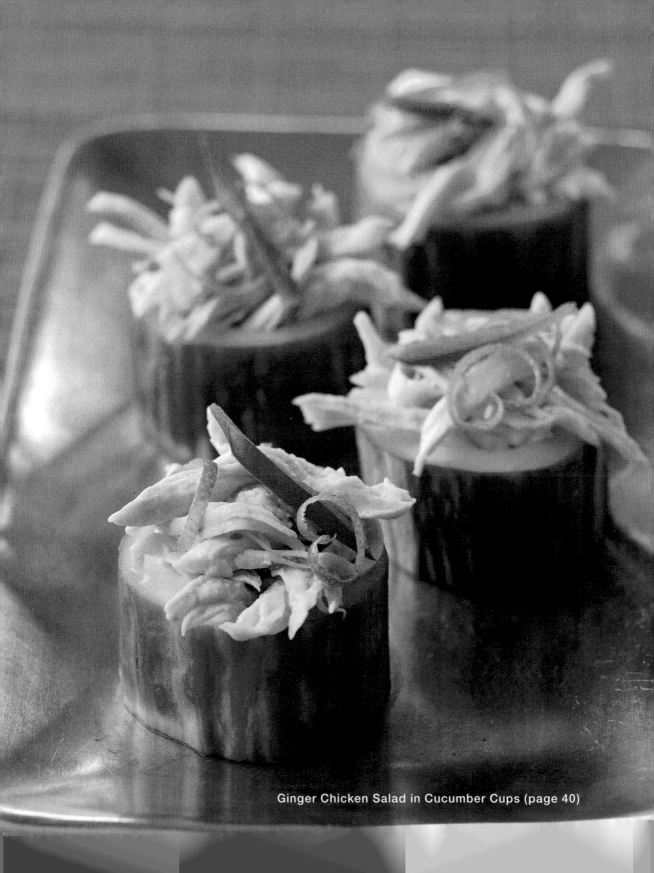

Ginger Chicken Salad in Cucumber Cups (page 40)

STARTERS, SNACKS, AND DRINKS

It seems counterintuitive that eating snacks (including healthy drinks) should be an important part of a weight loss program, but on the South Beach Diet adding healthful mini-meals between your main meals is essential for keeping blood sugar and cravings under control throughout the day.

Whether you're just beginning Phase 1 of the South Beach Diet or are continuing to work toward a healthy target weight on Phase 2, we don't ever want you to skip a meal or miss a snack. In addition, enjoying a filling starter before a main meal helps you feel fuller longer (which translates into not overeating at lunch and dinner).

Nearly all of the starters and snacks in this chapter travel well, so consider making big batches of our crispy adobo lentils or South Beach Diet snack mix to nibble on when energy flags. Or pack some deviled eggs or shrimp cocktail for a midafternoon pick-me-up. For other healthy grab-and-go snacks, see page 20.

Ginger Chicken Salad in Cucumber Cups

MAKES 16 cucumber cups (4 per serving)   HANDS-ON TIME: 20 minutes   TOTAL TIME: 30 minutes

Be sure to shred the chicken into very small pieces so that you can easily distribute the salad among the cucumber cups.

1 large (6-ounce) boneless, skinless chicken breast half

2 large English cucumbers (9 inches long)

1 teaspoon grated lime zest

2½ tablespoons fresh lime juice (1 large lime)

4 teaspoons canola oil or extra-virgin olive oil

1 teaspoon dark sesame oil

1 teaspoon minced peeled fresh ginger

Salt

Slivers of lime zest and red bell pepper, for garnish (optional)

Place the chicken breast in a small saucepan with just enough water to cover. Bring to a low boil over high heat. Reduce to a simmer and cook until mostly cooked through but still pink in the center, about 8 minutes. Remove the pan from the heat and let the chicken stand in the cooking water for 10 minutes.

Meanwhile, cut each cucumber crosswise into 8 rounds (about 1 inch thick). With a melon baller or small spoon, scoop out some of the seedy centers to make cups, taking care not to go through the bottoms.

In a medium bowl, stir together the lime zest, lime juice, canola oil, sesame oil, and ginger.

When cool enough to handle, pull the chicken into small shreds and add to the lime dressing. Stir to combine and season lightly with salt.

Fill the cucumber cups with chicken salad (a scant tablespoon each) and garnish with slivers of lime zest and bell pepper, if desired.

NUTRITION AT A GLANCE
Per cucumber cup: 29 calories, 2 g fat, 0 g saturated fat, 3 g protein, 1 g carbohydrate, 1 g fiber, 8 mg sodium

Broccoli, Pepper, and Cheese Bites

MAKES 16 pieces (2 per serving)   HANDS-ON TIME: 10 minutes   TOTAL TIME: 30 minutes

Serve these egg bites as part of a brunch or as a light lunch with a green salad. You can use frozen chopped kale instead of broccoli and any reduced-fat sharp cheese you prefer.

½ cup fat-free or 1% milk

⅓ cup part-skim ricotta cheese

2 tablespoons chickpea flour

6 large eggs

2 large egg whites (¼ cup)

¾ teaspoon salt

1 package (10 ounces) frozen chopped broccoli, thawed and well drained

1 jar (7 ounces) sliced roasted red peppers, drained

4 ounces shredded reduced-fat sharp Cheddar cheese (1 cup)

Heat the oven to 350°F. Lightly coat a 9 × 13-inch baking pan with cooking spray.

In a large bowl, whisk together the milk, ricotta, and flour until combined. Whisk in the eggs, egg whites, and salt until smooth. Stir in the broccoli, peppers, and cheese until well combined. Pour into the pan. Bake for 17 to 20 minutes, until set.

Cut into 16 rectangles and serve warm or at room temperature.

NUTRITION AT A GLANCE
Per piece: 71 calories, 4 g fat, 2 g saturated fat, 6 g protein, 3 g carbohydrate, 1 g fiber, 236 mg sodium

Cherry Tomato and Feta Crisps

MAKES 16 crisps (4 per serving)   HANDS-ON TIME: 10 minutes   TOTAL TIME: 30 minutes

There's no need to chop the garlic to flavor the oil for the crisps; just smash the clove with the flat side of a chef's knife, remove the peel, and toss into the olive oil. This recipe can easily be doubled or tripled for a crowd.

TOPPING

12 cherry tomatoes, halved

1 teaspoon extra-virgin olive oil

Salt and freshly ground black pepper

⅓ cup crumbled reduced-fat feta cheese

3 large black olives, pitted and slivered

Fresh rosemary sprigs, for garnish

CRISPS

1 large garlic clove, smashed and peeled

1 tablespoon extra-virgin olive oil

1 (8-inch) whole-wheat pita round

Salt and freshly ground black pepper

Heat the oven to 350°F.

For the topping: In a medium bowl, toss the tomatoes with the oil and salt and pepper to taste. Place the tomatoes on a baking sheet and bake, shaking the pan occasionally, for 10 to 15 minutes, or until softened.

While the tomatoes are baking, prepare the crisps: In a cup, stir the smashed garlic into the oil. Cut the pita into 8 even, double-layer triangles. Separate each triangle into 2 wedges. Place the pita wedges split-side up in a single layer on another baking sheet. Brush with the garlic oil and sprinkle lightly with salt and pepper. Bake the pita wedges for 7 minutes, or until crisp and golden.

To assemble: Top the crisps with the tomatoes, feta, and olives. Garnish with rosemary sprigs. Serve warm or at room temperature.

NUTRITION AT A GLANCE
Per crisp: 30 calories, 2 g fat, 0.7 g saturated fat, 1 g protein, 2 g carbohydrate, 0 g fiber, 76 mg sodium

TIPS: The pita crisps can be made 1 day ahead and stored in a tightly covered container at room temperature. You can roast the tomatoes up to 4 hours ahead of time and set aside, lightly covered, at room temperature until ready to use.

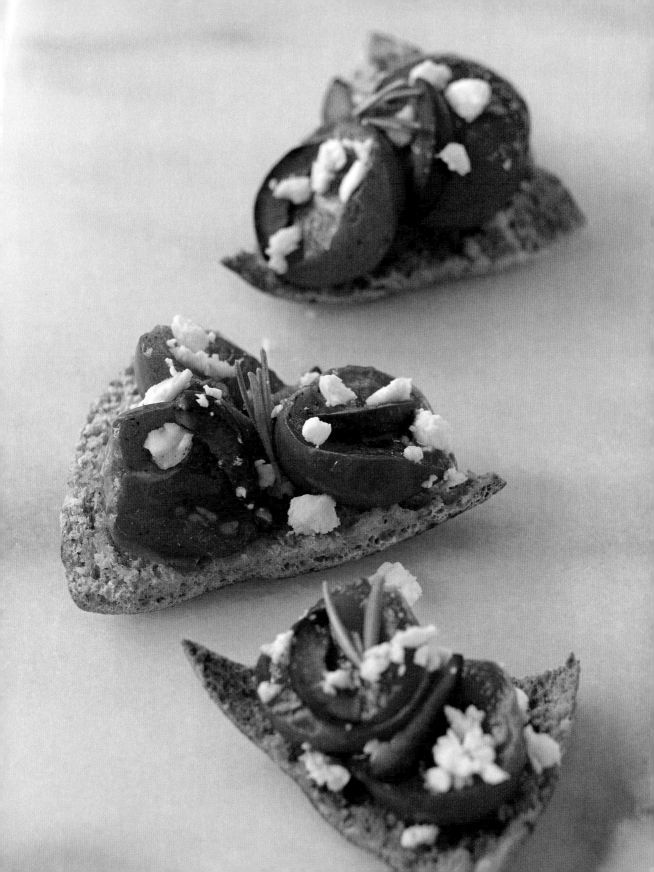

Lemony Stuffed Mushrooms

MAKES 12 stuffed mushrooms (3 per serving)   HANDS-ON TIME: 15 minutes
TOTAL TIME: 25 minutes

To get a head start on this already-quick appetizer, you can make the chickpea stuffing well in advance. Sturdy white mushrooms (called stuffer mushrooms on the packaging) are best here. Don't use Baby Bella or large cremini mushrooms because they don't hold their shape and you'll also have to scrape the gills out.

4 tablespoons fresh lemon juice

1 tablespoon extra-virgin olive oil

12 large white stuffer mushrooms (about 2½ inches), stems removed

1 can (15.5 ounces) chickpeas, rinsed and drained

3 tablespoons grated Parmesan cheese

2 teaspoons grated lemon zest

8 grape tomatoes, thinly sliced

Cracked black pepper

Heat the broiler.

In a large bowl, combine 2 tablespoons of the lemon juice and the oil. Add the mushroom caps, tossing to coat. Set aside to marinate while you make the stuffing.

In a mini food processor, combine the chickpeas, Parmesan, lemon zest, ¼ cup water, and remaining 2 tablespoons lemon juice. Process to a coarse purée.

Place the mushroom caps stemmed-side down on a rimmed baking sheet. Broil for 5 minutes, or until just beginning to release their liquid. Turn the mushrooms over and mound each with 2 tablespoons of the chickpea stuffing. Return to the broiler for 3 minutes to heat the stuffing.

Top each mushroom with tomato slices and a grinding of cracked pepper. Serve warm.

NUTRITION AT A GLANCE
Per mushroom: 46 calories, 2 g fat, 0.4 g saturated fat, 3 g protein, 5 g carbohydrate, 1 g fiber, 49 mg sodium

Shrimp Cocktail with Creamy Chipotle Sauce

**MAKES 4 servings (6 shrimp and ¼ cup sauce per serving)   HANDS-ON TIME: 25 minutes
TOTAL TIME: 25 minutes**

You can spend less time (but more money) if you buy shrimp that has already been peeled and deveined. Or save even more time (and spend the most money, of course) by buying cooked shrimp. If you do the latter, the recipe only takes 10 minutes total.

24 jumbo shrimp (about 1¼ pounds)	2 tablespoons mayonnaise
6 tablespoons tomato paste	2 tablespoons cider vinegar
3 tablespoons minced celery	¼ teaspoon chipotle chile powder
3 tablespoons minced sweet onion	

Peel and devein the shrimp. In a steamer, cook the shrimp for 6 to 8 minutes, or until pink and just opaque in the center.

Meanwhile, in a medium bowl, stir together the tomato paste, celery, onion, mayonnaise, vinegar, chipotle powder, and 5 tablespoons water. Serve 6 shrimp and ¼ cup chipotle sauce per person.

NUTRITION AT A GLANCE
Per serving: 119 calories, 6 g fat, 1 g saturated fat, 10 g protein, 6 g carbohydrate, 1 g fiber, 298 mg sodium

TIP: Be sure to buy a sweet variety of onion for this recipe. Vidalia, Walla Walla, or Maui are all good choices. Store the remaining onion in a resealable plastic bag in the fridge for up to 5 days.

15 MINUTE RECIPE

Smoked Salmon Canapés with Horseradish Cream

MAKES 18 canapés (3 per serving)   HANDS-ON TIME: 10 minutes   TOTAL TIME: 10 minutes

This elegant appetizer can be fine-tuned to suit your taste: Experiment with different whole-grain breads and try sprinkling with capers or lemon zest.

6 thin slices whole-grain bread

⅓ cup light or reduced-fat sour cream

1 tablespoon prepared horseradish

4 ounces smoked salmon slices, cut into 18 (1-inch-wide) strips

Black pepper

Fresh dill sprigs, for garnish

Using a 2-inch fluted round or other shaped pastry cutter, cut the bread slices into 18 rounds.

In a small bowl, combine the sour cream and horseradish. Spread each bread round with about 1 teaspoon of the mixture. Fold the salmon slices in half and place on top; garnish with a sprinkling of pepper and a dill sprig. Serve at room temperature.

NUTRITION AT A GLANCE

Per canapé: 51 calories, 2 g fat, 0.5 g saturated fat, 5 g protein, 4 g carbohydrate, 1 g fiber, 39 mg sodium

Chicken Tostaditas

MAKES 24 tostaditas (4 per serving)   HANDS-ON TIME: 25 minutes   TOTAL TIME: 25 minutes

Chipotle chiles, which lend their smoky flavor to these appetizers, are dried, smoked jalapeño peppers. They are typically found pickled and canned in a piquant adobo sauce in the Mexican food section of your supermarket. You can seed the chipotle or not before using, depending on how much heat you want. Place any unused chiles and adobo sauce in a plastic container and freeze for later use.

- 1 large (6-ounce) boneless, skinless chicken breast half
- 3 (8-inch) whole-wheat tortillas
- 3 teaspoons extra-virgin olive oil
- 2 garlic cloves, minced
- 1 cup tomatoes in purée
- 1 chipotle chile in adobo sauce, minced

- ½ teaspoon ground cumin
- ¼ teaspoon ground coriander
-   Salt
- 2 tablespoons reduced-fat sour cream
-   Fresh cilantro leaves, for garnish

Heat the oven to 400°F.

Place the chicken in a medium saucepan with cold water to cover. Bring to a simmer over high heat. Reduce the heat and let the chicken simmer for 8 minutes, or until cooked through and opaque on the inside. Cool the chicken in the cooking water, then drain and shred.

Meanwhile, brush the tops of the tortillas with 2 teaspoons of the oil. Cut each tortilla into 8 wedges and place on a baking sheet. Bake for 7 minutes, or until crisp and golden brown.

In a medium nonstick skillet, warm the remaining 1 teaspoon oil over medium-low heat. Add the garlic and cook, stirring, for 30 seconds. Add the tomatoes, chile, cumin, and coriander. Cook, stirring, until thickened, about 2 minutes. Transfer to a medium bowl and fold in the shredded chicken. Season with salt to taste.

Top each tortilla wedge with a spoonful of chicken mixture, then with a tiny dollop of sour cream. Garnish with a cilantro leaf. Serve warm or at room temperature.

NUTRITION AT A GLANCE
Per tostadita: 29 calories, 1 g fat, 0.2 g saturated fat, 2 g protein, 4 g carbohydrate, 0.5 g fiber, 71 mg sodium

TIP: You can prepare the chicken mixture 1 day ahead and refrigerate it until ready to use. Warm before using.

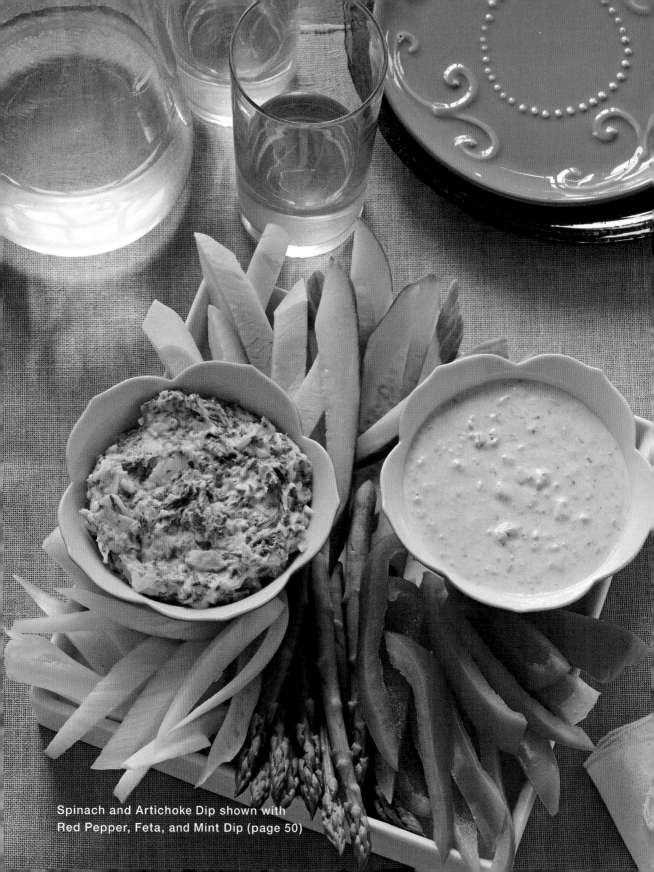

Spinach and Artichoke Dip shown with
Red Pepper, Feta, and Mint Dip (page 50)

Spinach and Artichoke Dip

MAKES 2⅔ cups   HANDS-ON TIME: 10 minutes   TOTAL TIME: 10 minutes

The popular artichoke dip that is a cocktail party staple typically calls for lots of high-fat mayonnaise. Our version uses part-skim ricotta and nutty Asiago cheese instead, which gives the dip a creamy, rich texture. Look for aged Asiago, which is easier to grate, and be sure to buy canned artichoke hearts rather than frozen or jarred marinated hearts (canned are more tender and flavorful than frozen, and far less fat-laden than those in the jar). Serve with Phase 1 veggies such as fennel, asparagus, red bell pepper, yellow squash, and cucumber.

1 package (10 ounces) frozen chopped spinach, thawed and squeezed dry	¾ cup part-skim ricotta cheese
	¾ teaspoon salt
1 can (13.75 ounces) artichoke hearts in water, drained	¼ teaspoon red pepper flakes
	Pinch nutmeg
1 tablespoon extra-virgin olive oil	½ cup grated aged Asiago cheese or Parmesan cheese
¼ teaspoon garlic powder	

In a food processor, combine the spinach, artichoke hearts, oil, and garlic powder. Pulse until finely chopped. Add the ricotta, salt, hot pepper flakes, and nutmeg. Pulse until smooth. Add the Asiago and pulse just until combined.

NUTRITION AT A GLANCE
Per tablespoon: 20 calories, 1 g fat, 0.5 g saturated fat, 1 g protein, 1 g carbohydrate, 0.5 g fiber, 69 mg sodium

**15
MINUTE
RECIPE**

Red Pepper, Feta, and Mint Dip

MAKES 1¾ cups   HANDS-ON TIME: 10 minutes   TOTAL TIME: 10 minutes

Serve this hearty, full-flavored dip with crudités of your choice. On Phase 2, it makes a great spread for a whole-wheat tortilla or pita.

1 jar (12 ounces) roasted red peppers, rinsed and drained

1 garlic clove, smashed and peeled

4 ounces reduced-fat cream cheese

4 ounces reduced-fat feta cheese

¼ cup nonfat (0%) plain Greek yogurt

3 tablespoons finely chopped fresh mint

1 tablespoon fresh lemon juice, or more to taste

1 tablespoon extra-virgin olive oil

Salt

In a food processor or blender, combine the peppers and garlic. Pulse until well blended. Add the cream cheese, feta, yogurt, mint, lemon juice, and oil. Process until blended but still thick. Add salt and additional lemon juice to taste. Serve at room temperature.

NUTRITION AT A GLANCE
Per tablespoon: 25 calories, 2 g fat, 1 g saturated fat, 2 g protein, 1 g carbohydrate, 0 g fiber, 104 mg sodium

TIP: The dip can be made up to 3 days ahead. Cover and refrigerate until ready to use.

Smoked-Trout Deviled Eggs

MAKES 12 halves (2 per serving)   **HANDS-ON TIME:** 10 minutes   **TOTAL TIME:** 20 minutes

This method of hard-boiling eggs makes for a soft, creamy yolk with no green border between the yolk and white. Hard-boiled eggs, still in their shells, will keep for a week in the refrigerator. The deviled eggs can be made several hours ahead, covered with plastic wrap, and refrigerated until ready to serve. Garnish with chives or scallions, if you prefer.

6 large eggs	1½ teaspoons Dijon mustard
2 ounces smoked trout, flaked, or 2 ounces smoked salmon, finely chopped	½ teaspoon salt
	⅛ teaspoon cayenne pepper
2 tablespoons mayonnaise	2 tablespoons chopped fresh dill

Place the eggs in a medium saucepan with cold water to cover. Bring to a boil over high heat. Remove from the heat, cover, and let stand for 12 minutes. Run the eggs under cold water to cool, then drain and peel.

While the eggs are standing, in a medium bowl, combine the smoked trout, mayonnaise, mustard, salt, and cayenne.

Cut the eggs in half lengthwise and, using a small spoon, scoop out the yolks. Add the yolks to the trout mixture and mash with a fork until well combined.

Spoon the mixture into the egg white halves and garnish with the dill.

NUTRITION AT A GLANCE
Per egg half: 62 calories, 5 g fat, 1 g saturated fat, 4 g protein, 0.5 g carbohydrate, 0 g fiber, 189 mg sodium

Spicy Lemon Edamame

MAKES 4 (1-cup) servings   HANDS-ON TIME: 5 minutes   TOTAL TIME: 20 minutes

Frozen edamame in the pod are easy to find in most supermarkets these days. This recipe will make them your new snack favorite on any phase of the diet. While the edamame are best served warm, they can also be chilled for a take-along snack. To save time, bring the water to a boil while you prep and measure the flavorful ingredients in the first step.

3 large garlic cloves, smashed and peeled

2 teaspoons coarse sea salt

2 large strips lemon zest, cut into thin slivers

½ teaspoon red pepper flakes

1 bag (16 ounces) frozen edamame in the pod

2 teaspoons fresh lemon juice

In a medium saucepan, combine 6 cups of water, the garlic, 1½ teaspoons of the sea salt, the lemon zest, and red pepper flakes. Cover and bring to a boil over high heat. Cook, partially covered, for 3 minutes to blend the flavors.

Add the frozen edamame. Return the water to a boil and cook, uncovered, for 3 minutes.

Drain well and transfer the edamame to a serving bowl. Discard the garlic. Toss the edamame with the lemon juice and remaining ½ teaspoon sea salt. Serve warm.

NUTRITION AT A GLANCE
Per serving: 79 calories, 2 g fat, 0 g saturated fat, 6 g protein, 9 g carbohydrate, 6 g fiber, 236 mg sodium

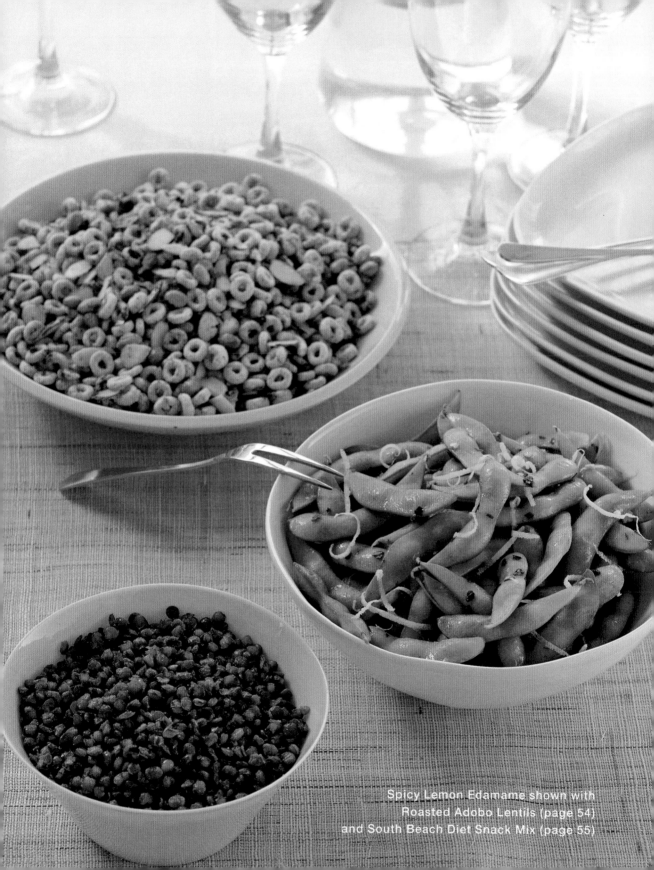

Spicy Lemon Edamame shown with
Roasted Adobo Lentils (page 54)
and South Beach Diet Snack Mix (page 55)

Roasted Adobo Lentils

MAKES 8 (¼-cup) servings   HANDS-ON TIME: 5 minutes   TOTAL TIME: 30 minutes

Here's a novel and healthy Phase 1 snack for those who love crunch but are tired of popcorn. Canned lentils are tossed with a little olive oil and adobo seasoning, then roasted. You can buy adobo seasoning, typically a mix of garlic powder, onion powder, black pepper, turmeric, oregano, and sometimes salt and dried citrus zest, at most supermarkets. You could just as easily toss the lentils with another seasoning mix of your choice or just plain sea salt.

 2 cans (15 ounces each) lentils, drained and rinsed
 2 tablespoons extra-virgin olive oil
 1½ teaspoons adobo seasoning

Heat the oven to 425°F. Using a paper towel, pat the lentils dry.

In a medium bowl, combine the lentils, oil, and adobo seasoning. Toss to coat well. Transfer to a large rimmed baking sheet, spreading the lentils out in a single layer.

Roast the lentils, shaking the baking sheet occasionally, for 20 to 25 minutes, or until lightly crisped. Cool briefly on the baking sheet before serving. Serve warm or at room temperature.

NUTRITION AT A GLANCE
Per serving: 92 calories, 3.5 g fat, 0.5 g saturated fat, 5 g protein, 10 g carbohydrate, 6 g fiber, 347 mg sodium

TIP: The lentils will keep for a couple of days in an airtight container at room temperature.

South Beach Diet Snack Mix

MAKES 8 (½-cup) servings   **HANDS-ON TIME: 5 minutes**   **TOTAL TIME: 25 minutes**

This healthy version of the famous fat-laden cereal "bridge mix" features natural almonds and roasted soy nuts and substitutes heart-healthy olive oil for the usual butter. For a spicy mix, simply add cayenne pepper to your taste.

- 3 cups regular toasted oat cereal
- ¾ cup grated Parmesan cheese (2 ounces)
- ⅔ cup sliced natural almonds
- 3 tablespoons extra-virgin olive oil
- ¾ teaspoon salt
- ½ cup roasted unsalted soy nuts

Heat the oven to 350°F.

In a large bowl, toss together the cereal, Parmesan, almonds, oil, and salt until well combined. Transfer to a large rimmed baking sheet and spread out in a single layer. Bake, stirring twice, for 20 minutes, or until the cereal is crisp and fragrant.

Transfer to a serving bowl and add the soy nuts, tossing to combine. Cool briefly and serve, or store in an airtight container at room temperature for a week.

NUTRITION AT A GLANCE
Per serving: 211 calories, 14 g fat, 2 g saturated fat, 10 g protein, 14 g carbohydrate, 3 g fiber, 408 mg sodium

15
MINUTE
RECIPE

Mocha Frappés

MAKES 2 (1-cup) servings   HANDS-ON TIME: 5 minutes   TOTAL TIME: 5 minutes

For this coffee shop favorite, we've used extra-strong coffee, which you can make by brewing 2 tablespoons of ground coffee for every cup of water. Be sure you do this a few hours ahead so there is time for the coffee to chill. This recipe makes enough for two drinks; to serve four, simply whip up another batch right away.

1 cup ice cubes

¾ cup very strong coffee, chilled

¾ cup fat-free or 1% milk

2 tablespoons granular sugar substitute

1 tablespoon sugar-free chocolate syrup

2 tablespoons no-sugar-added lite whipped topping

In a blender, combine the ice, coffee, milk, sugar substitute, and syrup. Blend on high speed until smooth. Pour into 2 tall glasses and add the whipped topping. Serve immediately.

NUTRITION AT A GLANCE
Per serving: 69 calories, 0.5 g fat, 0.5 g saturated fat, 4 g protein, 24 g carbohydrate, 0 g fiber, 63 mg sodium

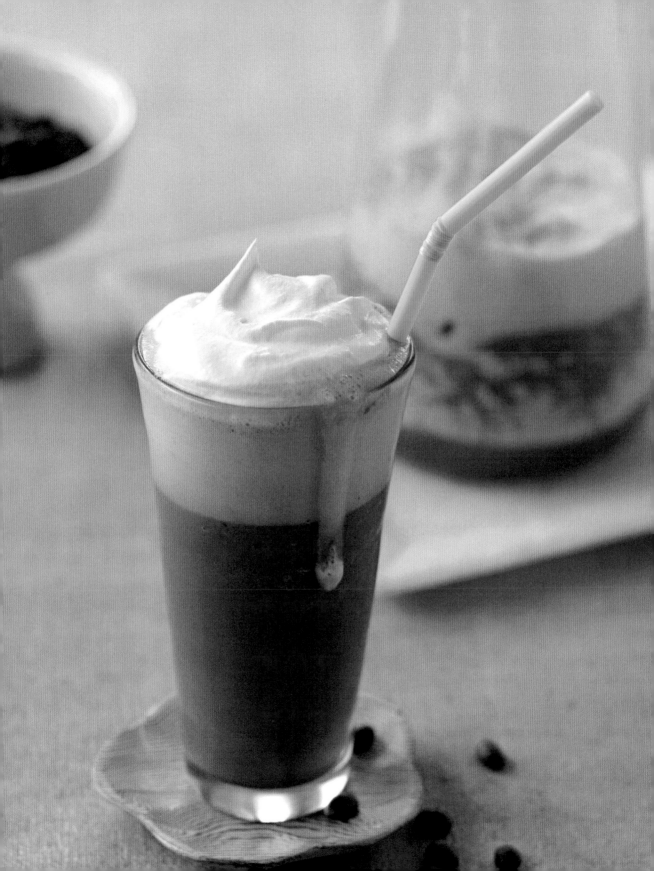

15
MINUTE
RECIPE

Triple Berry Coolers

MAKES 2 (1-cup) servings   HANDS-ON TIME: 5 minutes   TOTAL TIME: 5 minutes

A blend of vitamin-rich berries and calcium-loaded milk and yogurt, this healthful shake makes a great midmorning or midafternoon snack. For a change of pace, experiment with different yogurt flavors. The recipe serves two; you can easily cut it in half for one, or double it for more people (just make it in batches if you do).

¾ cup fresh or frozen raspberries

¾ cup fresh or frozen blueberries

¾ cup (6 ounces) artificially sweetened strawberry low-fat or nonfat yogurt

¼ cup fat-free or 1% milk

   Fresh berries, for garnish (optional)

In a blender or food processor, purée the berries. Add the yogurt and milk. Process until smooth. Pour into 2 tall glasses and garnish with additional fresh berries, if desired.

NUTRITION AT A GLANCE
Per serving: 116 calories, 0.5 g fat, 0 g saturated fat, 6 g protein, 24 g carbohydrate, 4 g fiber, 69 mg sodium

TIP: If you're using fresh berries and want a cooler beverage, simply add a few ice cubes when blending.

Spiced Chai Tea Smoothie

MAKES 1 (1-cup) serving   HANDS-ON TIME: 5 minutes   TOTAL TIME: 20 minutes

Enjoy this lightly spiced smoothie as an energizing midmorning snack. The lean protein from the milk and the tofu will help keep you satisfied until lunchtime. Look for chai tea bags where good teas are sold. You can easily double or triple the ingredients here, but it's best to process the smoothies one at a time.

½ cup fat-free or 1% milk

1 chai tea bag

½ cup lite silken tofu

1 tablespoon granular sugar substitute

¼ teaspoon pure almond extract

¼ teaspoon pure vanilla extract

6 to 8 ice cubes

Ground cinnamon, for garnish

In a glass measuring cup, warm the milk in a microwave oven for 1 minute. Add the tea bag and let steep for 10 minutes. Remove the tea bag and refrigerate the chai-milk for 5 minutes.

In blender or food processor, combine the chai-milk and tofu. Add the sugar substitute, almond and vanilla extracts, and ice. Process until the ice is crushed and the mixture is frothy. Sprinkle with cinnamon and serve chilled.

NUTRITION AT A GLANCE
Per serving: 69 calories, 1 g fat, 0 g saturated fat, 7 g protein, 9 g carbohydrate, 0 g fiber, 88 mg sodium

TIP: Look for lite silken tofu in the refrigerated section of your market; if it's unavailable, substitute low-fat or nonfat plain yogurt.

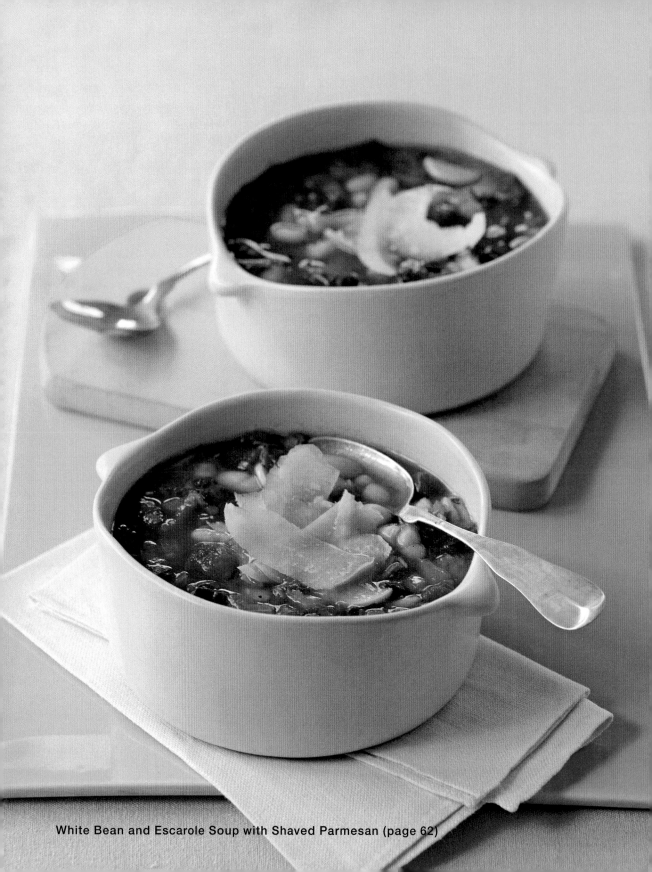

White Bean and Escarole Soup with Shaved Parmesan (page 62)

SOUPS AND SANDWICHES

We love soup and sandwiches on every phase of the South Beach Diet, and both are a boon to busy cooks. Soups lend themselves to freezing in small or large portions, and sandwiches can often be made ahead and refrigerated for quick meals at home or away.

Whether you enjoy it as a first course or as meal in itself (with or without a sandwich), soup is a great way to work more fiber (think vegetables, beans, and whole grains) and lean protein into your diet. Moreover, as you'll see from the recipes on the following pages, a sandwich needn't be synonymous with empty carbs and fatty luncheon meats. On Phase 1 you'll enjoy lean meat or poultry roll-ups with lettuce instead of bread, and on Phase 2 you'll find "sandwiches" in some fun new guises—try our squash pizzettes or shrimp-filled tortilla cones.

White Bean and Escarole Soup with Shaved Parmesan

MAKES 4 (1½-cup) servings   HANDS-ON TIME: 15 minutes   TOTAL TIME: 25 minutes

This soup freezes beautifully if you want to make it ahead (but don't add the cheese until just before you're ready to serve). Use a sharp knife to cut the escarole into 1-inch-wide ribbons. If you are watching your salt intake, you might want to use cooked dried white beans in this recipe (see Tip), rather than canned, which tends to be higher in sodium.

4   teaspoons extra-virgin olive oil

1   medium onion, finely chopped

3   garlic cloves, thinly sliced

½   teaspoon dried rosemary

1   can (15.5 ounces) white beans, drained and rinsed, or 1½ cups cooked dried beans

1   can (14.5 ounces) diced fire-roasted tomatoes, with juice

1¾   cups lower-sodium chicken broth

½   teaspoon salt

3   cups shredded escarole (5 ounces)

2   ounces Parmesan cheese, peeled into shards with a vegetable peeler

In a large saucepan, heat the oil over low heat. Add the onion, garlic, rosemary, and ⅓ cup water. Cook, stirring frequently, until the onion is tender, about 7 minutes.

Add the beans, tomatoes and their juice, broth, and salt. Bring to a boil. Reduce the heat and simmer 5 minutes longer for the flavors to blend.

Add the escarole and cook until wilted and tender, about 5 minutes.

Ladle the soup into 4 bowls, sprinkle evenly with the shaved Parmesan, and serve.

NUTRITION AT A GLANCE
Per serving: 241 calories, 9 g fat, 3 g saturated fat, 14 g protein, 27 g carbohydrate, 6 g fiber, 822 mg sodium

TIP: On a day when you have some time, soak and cook some dried white beans and then freeze them. They are great to have on hand for quick meals. One cup of dried beans will give you 2½ cups cooked beans.

Grilled Summer Squash Pizzettes

MAKES 4 pizzettes   HANDS-ON TIME: 30 minutes   TOTAL TIME: 30 minutes

Whole-wheat pita rounds make sturdy crusts for individual grilled pizzettes topped with summer squash and pesto. Feeling especially rushed? Top the pizzettes with thinly sliced fresh basil instead of pesto. If you prefer grilling outdoors, cover the grate with heavy-duty foil, and close the grill lid to melt the cheese.

PESTO

- ½ cup fresh basil leaves, coarsely chopped
- 2 tablespoons grated Parmesan cheese
- 1 tablespoon extra-virgin olive oil
- 1 tablespoon pine nuts

PIZZETTES

- 1 medium yellow squash
- 1 medium zucchini
- 2 teaspoons extra-virgin olive oil
  Salt and freshly ground black pepper
- 4 (8-inch) whole-wheat pita rounds
- ½ cup shredded part-skim mozzarella cheese (2 ounces)

For the pesto: In a blender or food processor, purée the basil, cheese, oil, and pine nuts until combined.

For the pizzettes: Halve the yellow squash and zucchini crosswise. Using a sharp knife or wide vegetable peeler, cut each half lengthwise into very thin ribbons.

In a large nonstick skillet, heat 1 teaspoon of the oil over medium-low heat. Add the yellow squash and zucchini ribbons and cook, stirring, until softened, about 6 minutes. Remove from the heat and season with salt and pepper.

Preheat a cast-iron grill pan. Brush the tops of the pitas with the remaining 1 teaspoon oil. Grill the pitas, oiled-side down, for 2 minutes, or until lightly browned. Remove to a work surface. Mound the squash ribbons atop the pita rounds, then dot each with 1 tablespoon pesto and sprinkle with 2 tablespoons mozzarella.

Grill the pitas for 4 minutes, or until the cheese melts. Serve hot.

NUTRITION AT A GLANCE
Per pizzette: 253 calories, 12 g fat, 3 g saturated fat, 11 g protein, 29 g carbohydrate, 5 g fiber, 377 mg sodium

TIP: The pesto can be made up to 7 days ahead and stored in an airtight container in the refrigerator. You'll have some left over from this recipe; use it to flavor sandwiches or whole-wheat pasta dishes.

15 MINUTE RECIPE

Lemon-Dill Soup with Scallops

MAKES 4 servings   **HANDS-ON TIME: 10 minutes**   **TOTAL TIME: 10 minutes**

Reminiscent of Greek avgolemono soup, this fast-to-prepare version adds scallops to the lemony broth.

4½ cups lower-sodium chicken broth

1 teaspoon grated lemon zest, plus more for garnish

¼ cup fresh lemon juice

4 scallions (white and tender green parts), thinly sliced

½ teaspoon salt

¾ pound medium-large sea scallops

⅓ cup minced fresh dill

Small fresh dill sprigs and lemon slices, for garnish (optional)

In a medium saucepan, combine the broth, lemon zest, lemon juice, scallions, and salt. Bring to a boil over medium-high heat and cook for 2 minutes to soften the scallions and flavor the broth.

Meanwhile, cut the scallops horizontally into thirds.

Add the scallops and dill to the soup and cook for 30 seconds. Remove the pan from the heat so scallops don't overcook.

Ladle the soup into 4 shallow bowls and garnish with dill sprigs and lemon slices and lemon zest, if using. Serve hot.

NUTRITION AT A GLANCE
Per serving: 101 calories, 1 g fat, 0 g saturated fat, 17 g protein, 6 g carbohydrate, 1 g fiber, 509 mg sodium

Variation: If you're on Phase 2, stir in 1 cup cooked quick-cooking barley when you add the scallops.

Per serving (with barley): 221 calories, 1 g fat, 0 g saturated fat, 21 g protein, 33 g carbohydrate, 4 g fiber, 509 mg sodium

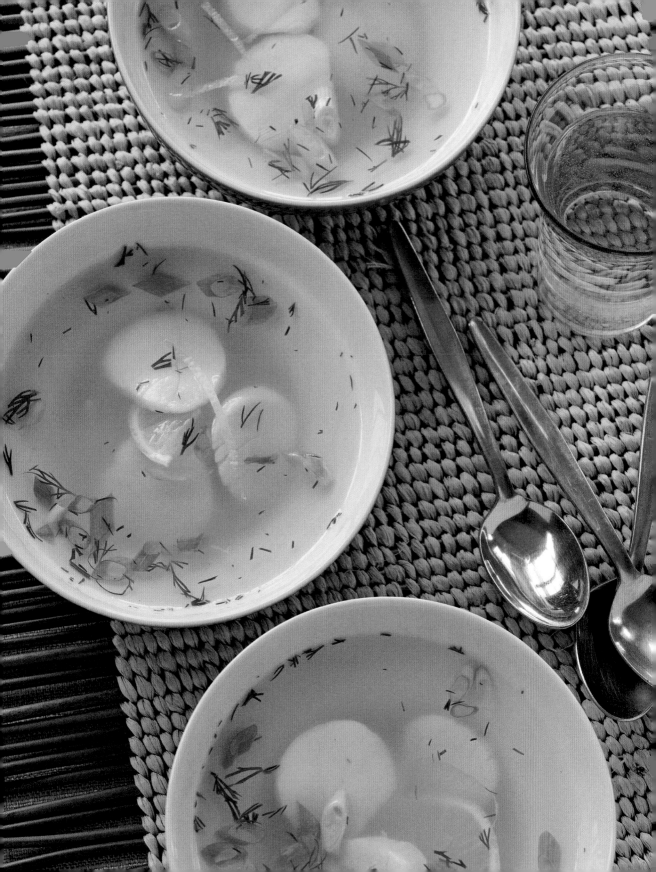

Japanese Turkey-Soba Soup

MAKES 4 (1¾-cup) servings   **HANDS-ON TIME: 10 minutes**   **TOTAL TIME: 20 minutes**

This satisfying soup lends itself to a number of variations. Instead of turkey, you could use 8 ounces baked tofu, cooked chicken breast, cooked chopped shrimp, or cooked pork loin. To save time, prep the bell pepper and turkey while the broth is coming to a boil.

5 cups lower-sodium chicken broth

2 teaspoons reduced-sodium soy sauce

1 garlic clove, minced

1 tablespoon slivered peeled fresh ginger

6 ounces soba noodles

1 small red bell pepper, finely slivered

8 ounces sliced lower-sodium deli turkey breast, slivered

2 cups baby spinach leaves (2 ounces)

1 teaspoon dark sesame oil

In a medium saucepan, bring the broth, soy sauce, garlic, and ginger to a boil over high heat. Add the soba and cook for the amount of time indicated in the package directions. Add the bell pepper for the last 2 minutes of cooking.

Remove the pan from the heat. Add the turkey and spinach. Push the spinach down into the broth and let sit for 30 seconds to wilt the spinach and heat the turkey through.

Stir in the sesame oil and serve hot.

NUTRITION AT A GLANCE
Per serving: 283 calories, 4 g fat, 1 g saturated fat, 23 g protein, 39 g carbohydrate, 1 g fiber, 554 mg sodium

Variations: For Phase 1 options, instead of using soba noodles, add ½ cup bean sprouts with the spinach or ½ cup very finely shredded cabbage with the bell pepper.

Per serving (with bean sprouts instead of soba): 149 calories, 4 g fat, 1 g saturated fat, 20 g protein, 10 g carbohydrate, 2 g fiber, 554 mg sodium

Per serving (with cabbage instead of soba): 142 calories, 4 g fat, 1 g saturated fat, 19 g protein, 9 g carbohydrate, 2 g fiber, 557 mg sodium

Asparagus Bisque

MAKES 4 (1-cup) servings   HANDS-ON TIME: 10 minutes   TOTAL TIME: 25 minutes

This recipe calls for chickpea flour, also known as garbanzo bean flour. It's an alternative to whole-wheat flour for thickening soups (and stews). You can find chickpea flour in most large supermarkets and online, or you can make your own (see Tip). Be sure to buy cut-up frozen asparagus rather than the more expensive spears, since the asparagus is going to be puréed anyway.

¼ cup sliced almonds	¼ teaspoon salt
¼ cup nonfat dry milk powder	Pinch cayenne pepper
2 tablespoons chickpea flour or whole-wheat flour	2 packages (10 ounces each) frozen cut-up asparagus spears
3 cups 1% or fat-free milk	2 wedges (¾ ounce each) light spreadable cheese
1 teaspoon dried tarragon	

Heat the oven to 350°F. Spread the almonds on a baking sheet and toast in the oven for 5 minutes, or until golden; set aside.

In a large saucepan, whisk together the dry milk and chickpea flour. Gradually whisk in the 1% milk until smooth. Cook over medium heat, whisking constantly, until the mixture is the consistency of heavy cream, about 5 minutes.

Whisk in the tarragon, salt, and cayenne. Add the asparagus and cook until tender, about 5 minutes. Transfer the soup, in batches, to a blender (or use an immersion blender) and purée until smooth. Return to the pan and bring to a simmer over low heat. Add the cheese and stir until melted. Ladle the soup into 4 bowls and sprinkle evenly with the almonds.

NUTRITION AT A GLANCE
Per serving: 189 calories, 6 g fat, 2 g saturated fat, 14 g protein, 20 g carbohydrate, 3 g fiber, 559 mg sodium

---

TIP: To make your own chickpea flour, rinse and drain canned chickpeas. Spread out on a baking sheet and leave out overnight to dry thoroughly. Process in a food processor until finely ground. Pass through a strainer and reprocess any lumps. Store in a resealable plastic bag in the freezer.

15 MINUTE RECIPE

Smoked Turkey Roll-Ups with Lemony Avocado Spread

MAKES 4 roll-ups   HANDS-ON TIME: 15 minutes   TOTAL TIME: 15 minutes

Wrap these delicious roll-ups individually in foil or plastic wrap and refrigerate overnight for a quick grab-and-go snack the following day. For a party presentation, tie the rolls with blanched chives. Remember that 2 tablespoons of this spread is equivalent to 2 tablespoons of an oil on all phases of the South Beach Diet.

½ avocado

2 tablespoons low-fat or nonfat plain yogurt

1 teaspoon grated lemon zest

1 tablespoon fresh lemon juice

Salt and freshly ground black pepper

¼ cup minced fresh chives

4 large buttercrunch or Boston lettuce leaves

½ pound thinly sliced smoked turkey

6 ounces thinly sliced reduced-fat Swiss cheese

4 long chives blanched in boiling water for 30 seconds (optional)

Scoop the avocado into a small bowl and, using a fork, mash with the yogurt, lemon zest, lemon juice, salt to taste, and a generous amount of black pepper. Stir in the minced chives and blend until the dressing is very smooth and spreadable.

Place a lettuce leaf on a work surface. Using one-fourth each of the turkey, cheese, and avocado mixture (about 2 tablespoons), place alternating slices of cheese and turkey on the leaf, spreading avocado mixture between layers as you go. Roll up the leaf and tie closed with a blanched chive, if using.

Make 3 more roll-ups using the remaining ingredients.

NUTRITION AT A GLANCE
Per roll-up: 180 calories, 8 g fat, 4 g saturated fat, 27 g protein, 3 g carbohydrate, 0.5 g fiber, 425 mg sodium

TIP: To use the entire avocado (so the leftover half doesn't turn brown), make a double batch of this spread. It will keep in the refrigerator for a few days. Enjoy it with crudités, or whole-wheat crackers if you're on Phase 2.

Two-Mushroom Cauliflower Soup

MAKES 4 (1¾-cup) servings   HANDS-ON TIME: 20 minutes   TOTAL TIME: 30 minutes

Soak the porcini as long as possible to extract the maximum flavor. If you have an immersion blender, it works just fine for this recipe and will save you some time. A squeeze or two of lemon brings out the mushroomy flavor.

¼ ounce dried porcini mushrooms (about ⅓ cup)

3½ cups lower-sodium chicken broth

1 tablespoon extra-virgin olive oil

8 ounces cremini mushrooms, quartered

1 small onion, thinly sliced

2 garlic cloves, minced

1 package (20 ounces) frozen cauliflower florets

¾ teaspoon salt

¼ teaspoon freshly ground black pepper

4 tablespoons reduced-fat sour cream

¼ teaspoon grated nutmeg

1 large lemon, cut into 8 wedges, for serving

In a small saucepan, bring the porcini mushrooms and ½ cup of the broth to a simmer over high heat. Remove from the heat and set aside to allow the mushrooms to soften while you prepare and cook the vegetables.

In a medium nonstick saucepan, heat the oil over medium heat. Add the cremini mushrooms, onion, and garlic. Cook, stirring often, until softened, about 3 minutes.

Meanwhile, place the frozen cauliflower in a strainer and run under hot water to warm a bit.

Add the remaining 3 cups broth to the soup. Drain the porcini in a strainer held over the saucepan so the soaking liquid is added to the soup. Add the cauliflower, salt, and pepper and bring to a boil over high heat. Reduce the heat and simmer for 1 minute to heat the cauliflower through.

Meanwhile, cut the porcini into slivers.

Transfer the hot soup in batches to a blender (or use an immersion blender) and purée until smooth. Whisk in 3 tablespoons of the sour cream and the nutmeg.

Ladle the soup into 4 bowls and top each with some slivered porcini and 1 scant teaspoon sour cream. Serve with lemon wedges for squeezing.

NUTRITION AT A GLANCE

Per serving: 165 calories, 7 g fat, 2 g saturated fat, 11 g protein, 17 g carbohydrate, 5 g fiber, 554 mg sodium

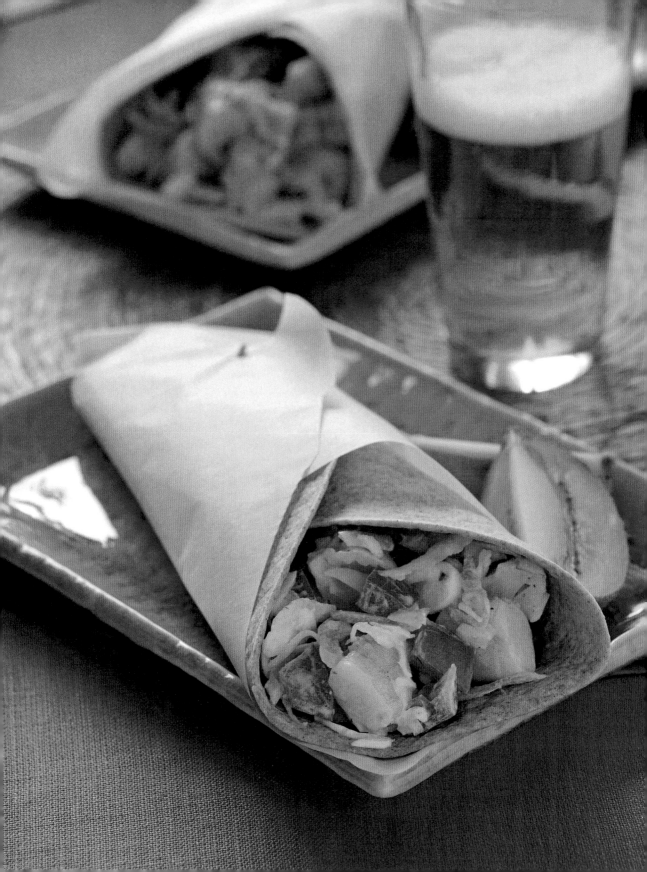

Shrimp Cones

MAKES 4 servings   HANDS-ON TIME: 15 minutes   TOTAL TIME: 20 minutes

Serving shrimp salad in a tortilla cone is a nice change from a whole-wheat bun. You can make this quick recipe even speedier by buying cooked shrimp.

¾ pound peeled and deveined large shrimp

2 tablespoons mayonnaise

1 tablespoon cider vinegar

1 tablespoon low-fat plain yogurt

¼ teaspoon freshly ground black pepper

1 cup coleslaw mix

2 plum tomatoes, coarsely chopped

4 (8-inch) whole-wheat tortillas

4 teaspoons Dijon mustard

In a steamer, bring about 1 inch of water to a boil (do not add shrimp until the water is boiling). Add the shrimp, cover, and cook for 6 to 8 minutes, until they turn pink and are just opaque in the center. Rinse under cold water to cool, then coarsely chop.

While the shrimp are cooking, in a medium bowl, combine the mayonnaise, vinegar, yogurt, and pepper. Add the coleslaw mix and tomatoes and toss well.

Add the shrimp to the cabbage mixture and toss.

Spread a tortilla with 1 teaspoon mustard. Roll into a cone shape and fill with 1 cup of the shrimp mixture. Repeat to make 3 more cones.

NUTRITION AT A GLANCE
Per serving: 232 calories, 8 g fat, 1 g saturated fat, 21 g protein, 25 g carbohydrate, 3 g fiber, 463 mg sodium

Variation: For a Phase 1 recipe, omit the tortillas and shred your own cabbage instead of using coleslaw mix, which typically has shredded carrots in it.

Per serving (without tortilla): 158 calories, 7 g fat, 1 g saturated fat, 18 g protein, 4 g carbohydrate, 1 g fiber, 291 mg sodium

Smoky Lentil Soup

MAKES 4 (1¾-cup) servings   HANDS-ON TIME: 10 minutes   TOTAL TIME: 25 minutes

The smokiness in this hearty soup comes from chile powder. Chipotle powder is a little hotter and smokier than ancho powder, so use chipotle when you want a spicier soup. If you have a little extra time, cook the lentils from scratch. One cup of dried lentils makes 2½ cups cooked (the equivalent of the two cans used here).

4 teaspoons extra-virgin olive oil

1 medium carrot, halved lengthwise and thinly sliced

3 scallions, thinly sliced

2 garlic cloves, thinly sliced

1 teaspoon ancho chile powder or chipotle chile powder

2 cans (15 ounces each) lentils, drained and rinsed

1 can (14.5 ounces) diced tomatoes, with juice

1¾ cups lower-sodium chicken broth

2 ounces thinly sliced smoked ham, coarsely chopped (½ cup)

In a large saucepan, heat the oil over medium heat. Add the carrot and cook, stirring frequently, until tender, about 5 minutes.

Stir in the scallions, garlic, and chile powder and cook for 1 minute. Add the lentils, tomatoes and their juice, the broth, and ham. Bring to a boil. Reduce the heat and simmer for 10 minutes for the flavors to develop.

Ladle the soup into 4 bowls and serve hot.

NUTRITION AT A GLANCE
Per serving: 225 calories, 6 g fat, 1 g saturated fat, 15 g protein, 28 g carbohydrate, 12 g fiber, 566 mg sodium

"Tortilla" Soup

MAKES 4 servings   **HANDS-ON TIME: 15 minutes**   **TOTAL TIME: 25 minutes**

Here's a richly flavored, quick-cooking Southwestern-style soup that tastes like you simmered it for hours. Our healthy Phase 1 recipe has all the elements of a traditional tortilla soup—except the fried tortilla strips.

1 tablespoon extra-virgin olive oil

½ medium red onion, finely chopped

3 garlic cloves, minced

1 teaspoon ground cumin

Pinch cayenne pepper

3½ cups lower-sodium chicken broth

1 can (14.5 ounces) diced tomatoes, with juice

¾ pound boneless, skinless chicken breasts, cut into ½-inch cubes

3 tablespoons fresh lime juice

Salt and freshly ground black pepper

¼ cup chopped fresh cilantro

In a medium saucepan, heat the oil over medium-low heat. Add the onion, garlic, cumin, and cayenne. Cook, stirring often, until the onion is softened, about 4 minutes.

Add the broth and tomatoes and their juice. Bring to a boil. Reduce the heat and simmer for 5 minutes.

Add the chicken and return to a simmer. Cook until the chicken is cooked through, about 4 minutes.

Remove the pan from the heat and stir in the lime juice. Season with salt and pepper to taste. Ladle the soup into 4 bowls and sprinkle with the cilantro.

NUTRITION AT A GLANCE
Per serving: 180 calories, 5 g fat, 1 g saturated fat, 24 g protein, 8 g carbohydrate, 1 g fiber, 395 mg sodium

Open-Face Stack Sandwiches

MAKES 4 sandwiches   HANDS-ON TIME: 20 minutes   TOTAL TIME: 20 minutes

For these fun sandwiches, choose multigrain English muffins with 2.5 or 3 grams of fiber per muffin half. Use a light hand when rubbing the muffins with the raw garlic; a little goes a long way! On Phase 3, enjoy two stacks if you like.

2 multigrain English muffins	1 cup baby spinach leaves (1 ounce)
1 large garlic clove, halved	8 thin slices (5 ounces) lower-sodium deli turkey breast, folded into quarters
½ avocado	
2 teaspoons fresh lime juice	4 thin slices red onion
¼ teaspoon chili powder	4 slices (2 ounces) reduced-fat provolone cheese, folded into quarters
Pinch salt	
1 jar (6 ounces) roasted red peppers, drained and rinsed	

Split the English muffins and toast. Lightly rub the cut sides with the cut garlic clove.

Meanwhile, scoop the avocado into a small bowl. With a fork, mash with the lime juice, chili powder, and salt.

Cut four 2-inch squares of roasted peppers and cut any remainder into thin strips.

For each sandwich, top an English muffin half with the following: 1 tablespoon avocado mixture, a couple spinach leaves, 1 slice turkey, 1 slice onion, a roasted pepper square, 1 slice provolone, another slice of turkey, some more spinach leaves, and strips of roasted pepper.

NUTRITION AT A GLANCE
Per sandwich: 206 calories, 7 g fat, 2 g saturated fat, 15 g protein, 22 g carbohydrate, 4 g fiber, 540 mg sodium

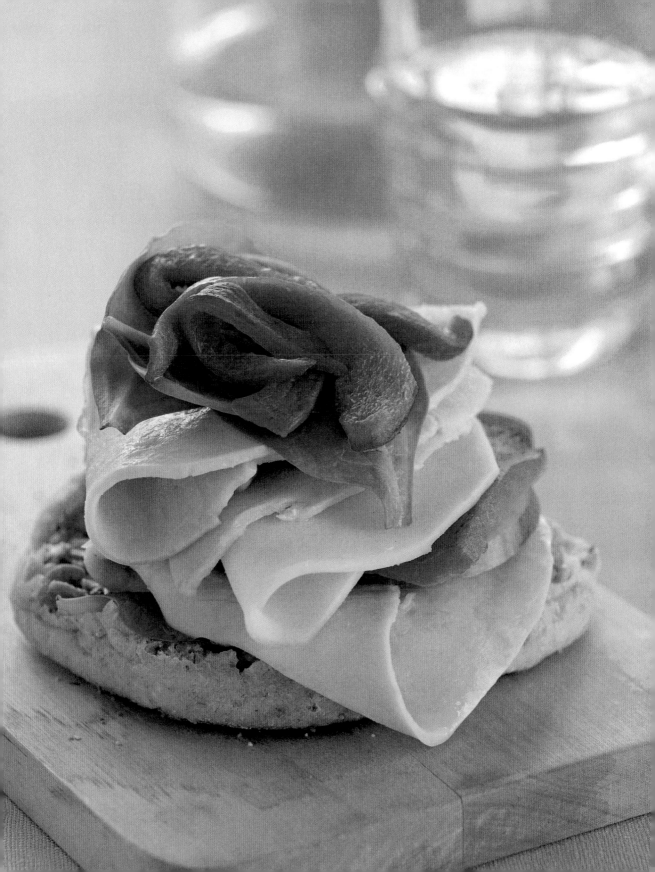

Spiced Sweet Potato–Tomato Soup

MAKES 4 (1¼-cup) servings HANDS-ON TIME: 15 minutes TOTAL TIME: 30 minutes

This hearty soup uses delicious, healthy pumpkin seeds as a garnish. You can purchase hulled pumpkin seeds already toasted, but for maximum flavor it's best to toast your own. The cheese adds creaminess to the soup with very little fat.

1¼ pounds sweet potatoes, peeled and cut into ½-inch cubes

¼ cup hulled pumpkin seeds (1 ounce)

1 can (14.5 ounces) spicy diced tomatoes, with juice

1¼ cups lower-sodium chicken broth

3 wedges (¾ ounce each) light spreadable cheese

½ teaspoon ground coriander

¼ teaspoon ground cinnamon

¼ teaspoon salt

In a steamer, cook the sweet potatoes for 10 to 15 minutes, or until tender when pierced with the tip of a knife.

Meanwhile, in a small ungreased skillet, toast the pumpkin seeds over medium heat, tossing occasionally, until lightly browned and puffed up a bit, 3 to 5 minutes. Scrape onto a plate to stop the cooking.

Transfer the hot sweet potatoes to a food processor. Add the tomatoes and their juice, the broth, cheese, coriander, cinnamon, and salt. Purée until smooth.

Ladle the soup into 4 bowls and sprinkle each with 1 tablespoon toasted pumpkin seeds. Serve warm.

NUTRITION AT A GLANCE
Per serving: 200 calories, 6 g fat, 2 g saturated fat, 8 g protein, 30 g carbohydrate, 4 g fiber, 707 mg sodium

Asian Beef in Lettuce Cups

MAKES 4 servings (3 lettuce cups per serving)   **HANDS-ON TIME: 5 minutes**
TOTAL TIME: 15 minutes

Lettuce leaves make the perfect "bread" for these Phase 1 "sandwiches." If you prefer, you can substitute snow peas for the snap peas and any type of sprouts for the mung bean sprouts.

2 tablespoons reduced-sodium soy sauce	8 ounces sugar snap peas, strings removed
1 tablespoon dark sesame oil	2 cups shredded radicchio (from half a small head)
½ teaspoon ground ginger	2 cups mung bean sprouts
1 pound beef sirloin, cut into ½-inch-wide strips	2 tablespoons rice vinegar
1 teaspoon extra-virgin olive oil	12 Boston lettuce leaves

In a large bowl, whisk together the soy sauce, sesame oil, and ginger. Add the beef and toss to coat.

In a large nonstick skillet, heat the olive oil over medium-high heat. Add half the beef and cook until browned, about 1 minute on each side. With a slotted spoon, transfer to a large bowl. Repeat with the remaining beef.

In a small pan of boiling water, cook the snap peas for 30 seconds. Drain, rinse under cold water, and drain again.

Transfer the snap peas to the bowl with beef. Add the radicchio, sprouts, and vinegar and toss well.

Divide the beef mixture evenly among the lettuce leaves and serve.

NUTRITION AT A GLANCE
Per serving: 255 calories, 11 g fat, 3 g saturated fat, 28 g protein, 10 g carbohydrate, 3 g fiber, 528 mg sodium

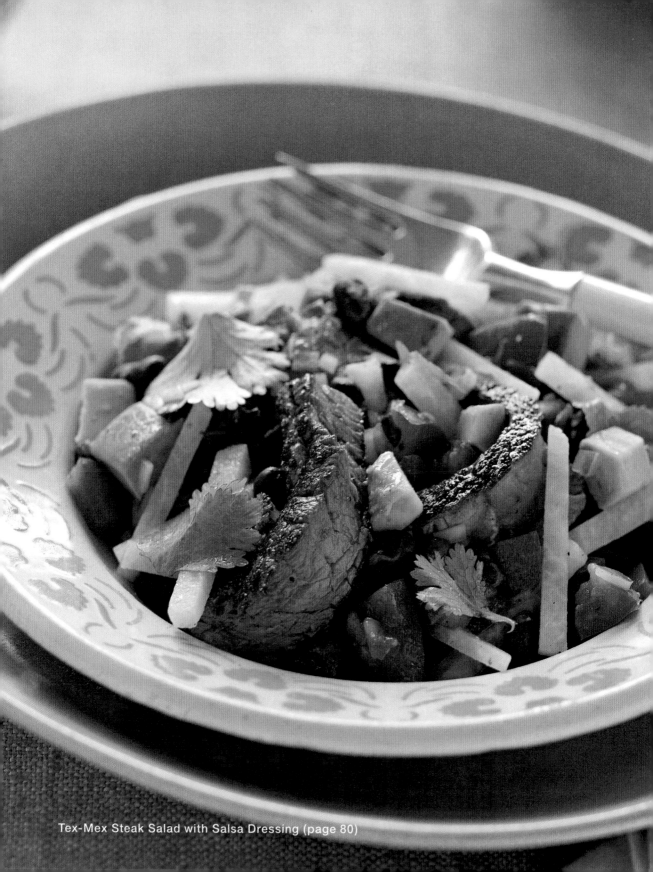

Tex-Mex Steak Salad with Salsa Dressing (page 80)

MAIN-DISH SALADS

Main-dish salads typically take time because of all the chopping required. But today salad-making no longer needs to be a tedious, labor-intensive process, thanks to the endless number of prewashed lettuce mixes, pre-chopped vegetables, and prepared low-sugar dressings available in every supermarket. Just add some chicken, turkey, seafood, reduced-fat cheese, beans, or tofu, and you've got a healthy and filling lunch or dinner.

As you review the main-course salad recipes on the following pages, remember that you can easily double or triple the amounts, or halve them to make a dinner for two. Also consider mixing and matching the flavorful dressings and making extra to store in the fridge for another healthy salad meal.

No time to cook? Enjoy one of the no-cook salads on page 18.

Tex-Mex Steak Salad with Salsa Dressing

MAKES 4 (1½-cup) servings HANDS-ON TIME: 10 minutes TOTAL TIME: 20 minutes

This quick beefy salad calls for jícama, a nonstarchy tuber that is crisp and juicy. You can find jícama in the produce department of the supermarket, either in the Latin American section or with the potatoes and onions. A jícama can weigh anywhere from ½ pound to 5 pounds; look for a small one that is firm and heavy for its size. Use a vegetable peeler (see page 13 for a good one) or paring knife to remove the brown papery skin before cutting into matchstick-size pieces (julienne).

1½ teaspoons ground coriander

1 teaspoon ground cumin

¾ teaspoon dried oregano

¾ teaspoon salt

1 (1¼-pound) sirloin steak

4 teaspoons extra-virgin olive oil

1 cup whole fresh cilantro leaves

1 cup julienned jícama

2 plum tomatoes, diced

⅓ cup prepared no-sugar-added black bean salsa

2 tablespoons fresh lime juice

½ avocado, cut into ½-inch dice

In a small bowl, stir together the coriander, cumin, oregano, and salt. Rub the mixture into both sides of the steak.

In a medium skillet, heat 1 teaspoon of the oil over medium-high. Add the steak and cook for 2 to 3 minutes per side for medium-rare (longer for more well done). Transfer to a cutting board and let stand for 5 minutes.

Meanwhile, in a large bowl, combine the cilantro, jícama, tomatoes, salsa, lime juice, and remaining 3 teaspoons oil.

Thinly slice the steak, add to the bowl, and toss to combine. Divide the salad evenly among 4 plates and scatter the avocado evenly over the tops.

NUTRITION AT A GLANCE
Per serving: 295 calories, 14 g fat, 4 g saturated fat, 33 g protein, 9 g carbohydrate, 4 g fiber, 608 mg sodium

California Turkey Salad with Fresh Tomato-Lime Dressing

MAKES 4 servings   HANDS-ON TIME: 15 minutes   TOTAL TIME: 15 minutes

For this salad you will need to buy one or two large pieces (not sliced) smoked turkey from the deli so you can cut it into cubes. Smoked turkey can be quite high in sodium, so if you are concerned about your salt intake, use regular roast turkey (or even crabmeat) instead.

- 5 plum tomatoes (1¼ pounds)
- 2 tablespoons fresh lime juice
- 2 tablespoons extra-virgin olive oil
  Salt
- 1 head romaine lettuce, thinly sliced crosswise (8 cups)
- ¾ pound lower-sodium smoked turkey, in one piece, cut into ½-inch cubes
- 4 ounces part-skim mozzarella cheese, cut into ½-inch cubes
- 1 avocado, diced

Cut 2 of the plum tomatoes into thin wedges and set aside.

Quarter the remaining 3 tomatoes and place in a food processor along with the lime juice and oil. Process to a smooth purée. Season with salt to taste.

Divide the lettuce among 4 plates. For each salad, drizzle the lettuce with 1 tablespoon dressing and top with one-fourth each of the turkey, mozzarella, avocado, and tomato wedges. Drizzle each salad with 1 tablespoon dressing and serve.

NUTRITION AT A GLANCE

Per serving: 315 calories, 19 g fat, 5 g saturated fat, 29 g protein, 11 g carbohydrate, 5 g fiber, 721 mg sodium

Seven-Vegetable Salad

MAKES 4 servings   HANDS-ON TIME: 20 minutes   TOTAL TIME: 20 minutes

In this colorful version of a chopped salad, shredded vegetables are tossed with a tangy lemon vinaigrette. For a perfect take-along lunch, pack the dressing in a separate container and dress the salad just before eating. Really pressed for time? Use a prepared no-sugar-added dressing of your choice.

4 medium asparagus spears	1 tablespoon fresh lemon juice
1 large carrot, halved lengthwise	1 tablespoon white wine vinegar
1 small zucchini, quartered lengthwise	Salt and freshly ground black pepper
4 Belgian endive leaves	1½ cups canned chickpeas or cannellini beans, drained and rinsed
½ medium red bell pepper	
10 sugar snap peas (strings removed) or green beans	3 tablespoons reduced-fat goat cheese
2 tablespoons extra-virgin olive oil	½ cup pea shoots or alfalfa sprouts

Insert the shredding disk in a food processor. With the motor running, drop the asparagus, carrot, and zucchini through the feed tube to shred. With a sharp knife, thinly slice the endive, bell pepper, and snap peas.

In a large serving bowl, whisk together the oil, lemon juice, vinegar, and salt and pepper to taste. Add all the vegetables and the chickpeas and toss until thoroughly coated. Season to taste with additional salt and pepper.

Mound the salad onto 4 plates, dot evenly with the goat cheese, and sprinkle with the pea shoots.

NUTRITION AT A GLANCE
Per serving: 190 calories, 10 g fat, 2 g saturated fat, 8 g protein, 20 g carbohydrate, 6 g fiber, 160 mg sodium

---

TIP: If you don't have a food processor, a sturdy vegetable peeler will work just fine for shredding the vegetables. While you're at it, you might as well shred extra, since the vegetables will keep for 2 days in a covered container in the fridge.

Cook Once, Eat Twice

Double the recipe and add tuna to the extra for a heartier salad.

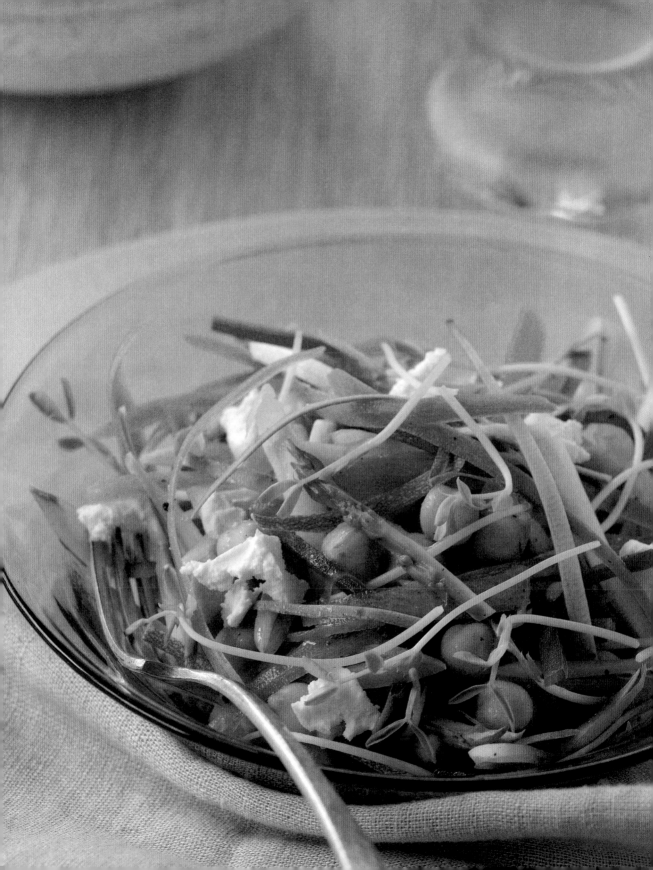

Beef and Broccoli Salad with Mustard Vinaigrette

MAKES 4 (2-cup) servings   HANDS-ON TIME: 15 minutes   TOTAL TIME: 25 minutes

Take advantage of the supermarket's precut produce for this recipe. Already cut-up broccoli will save you a few minutes of prep time.

- ¼ cup extra-virgin olive oil
- 3 tablespoons red wine vinegar
- 4 teaspoons Dijon mustard
- ½ teaspoon dried tarragon
- ¼ teaspoon salt
- 1 tablespoon nonpareil capers, drained and rinsed (optional)

- 1 (1-pound) well-trimmed sirloin steak
- 4 cups small broccoli florets (10 ounces)
- 2 medium yellow bell peppers, cut into ½-inch squares

Heat the broiler. Or heat a grill to medium-high.

In a large bowl, whisk together the oil, vinegar, 2 teaspoons of the mustard, the tarragon, and salt. Stir in the capers, if using.

Brush both sides of the beef with the remaining 2 teaspoons mustard. Broil or grill 6 inches from the heat for 5 minutes per side for medium-rare. Let the beef stand for 5 minutes before cutting across the grain into ½-inch-thick slices. Then cut the slices crosswise into 1-inch squares, reserving any juices that accumulate.

Meanwhile, in a steamer, cook the broccoli for 3 minutes until just barely tender. Add the hot broccoli to the bowl of dressing along with the bell peppers and stir to combine. Stir in the beef and beef juices. Serve warm, at room temperature, or chilled.

NUTRITION AT A GLANCE
Per serving: 331 calories, 22 g fat, 5 g saturated fat, 23 g protein, 10 g carbohydrate, 3 g fiber, 346 mg sodium

Cajun Salmon Salad

MAKES 4 servings   HANDS-ON TIME: 5 minutes   TOTAL TIME: 15 minutes

**15
MINUTE
RECIPE**

Make sure to buy salmon fillets with the skin on; the skin helps to preserve moistness when roasting. Use a thin metal spatula to lift the salmon off the baking sheet and the skin will stay behind. By purchasing "salad cut" hearts of palm you avoid any chopping when prepping this quick dish.

1 teaspoon paprika	2 tablespoons fresh lemon juice
½ teaspoon dried oregano	2 teaspoons extra-virgin olive oil
¼ teaspoon dried thyme	1 can (14 ounces) salad cut hearts of palm, drained and rinsed
⅛ teaspoon cayenne pepper	
¼ teaspoon salt	8 cups baby arugula (about 6 ounces)
4 (6-ounce) salmon fillets, skin on	

Heat the oven to 450°F. Line a rimmed baking sheet with foil.

In a small bowl, stir together the paprika, oregano, thyme, cayenne, and ⅛ teaspoon of the salt. Rub the mixture into the skinless side of each salmon fillet. Place the salmon on the baking sheet skin-side down. Roast for about 10 minutes, until just opaque throughout and the fish just flakes when tested with a fork.

Meanwhile, in a large bowl, whisk together the lemon juice, oil, and remaining ⅛ teaspoon salt. Add the hearts of palm and arugula and toss to coat.

Divide the arugula mixture among 4 plates, place a warm salmon fillet on top of each, and serve.

NUTRITION AT A GLANCE
Per serving: 365 calories, 22 g fat, 4 g saturated fat, 37 g protein, 6 g carbohydrate, 2 g fiber, 559 mg sodium

Cook Once, Eat Twice

Cook a double batch of the salmon and turn the extra into a completely different salmon salad by adding capers, sun-dried tomatoes, a little mayo, and a hard-boiled egg.

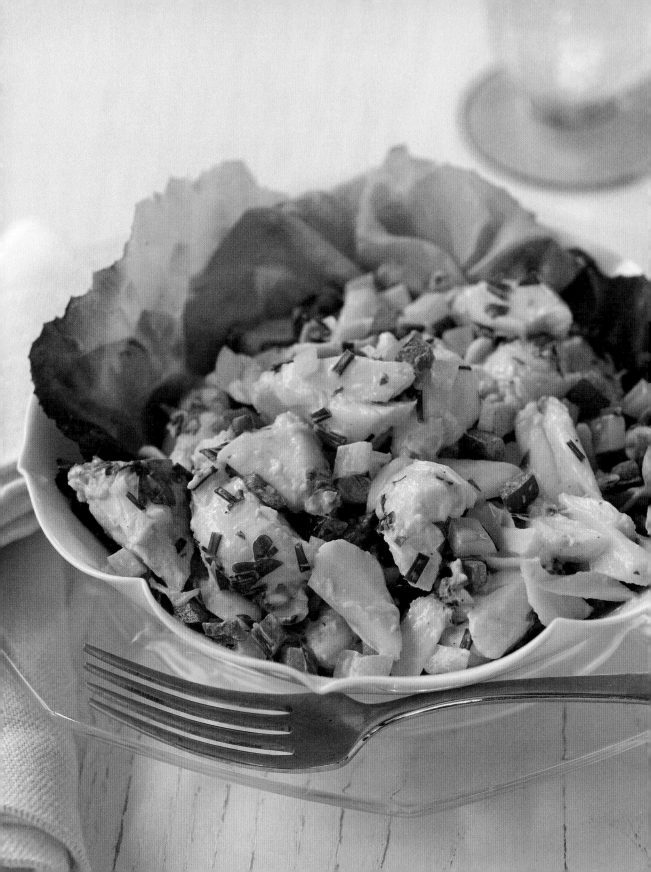

Confetti Crab Salad

MAKES 4 servings   HANDS-ON TIME: 15 minutes   TOTAL TIME: 15 minutes

15 MINUTE RECIPE

Here's a fresh change from tuna salad, made colorful and healthy with the addition of vitamin C–rich bell peppers. Be sure to pick over the crabmeat to remove any small bits of cartilage. If you like, use kitchen shears to snip the chives.

¼ cup mayonnaise

2 tablespoons fresh lemon juice

2 teaspoons Dijon mustard

1 pound jumbo lump crabmeat

1 medium red bell pepper, diced

1 medium yellow bell pepper, diced

¼ cup chopped fresh chives

¼ cup chopped fresh parsley

Salt and freshly ground black pepper

8 cups baby salad greens

In a serving bowl, combine the mayonnaise, lemon juice, and mustard. Fold in the crabmeat, bell peppers, chives, and parsley. Season with salt and pepper to taste.

Divide the salad greens among 4 salad bowls. Spoon the crab salad over the greens and serve.

NUTRITION AT A GLANCE

Per serving: 276 calories, 13 g fat, 2 g saturated fat, 29 g protein, 8 g carbohydrate, 3 g fiber, 594 mg sodium

TIP: Make the salad up to 1 day ahead and refrigerate, tightly covered.

Chicken, Mango, and Sugar Snap Pea Salad

MAKES 4 servings   **HANDS-ON TIME:** 10 minutes   **TOTAL TIME:** 25 minutes

Poaching the chicken keeps it moist without any added fat. For maximum flavor, serve the salad at room temperature.

- 3 (6-ounce) boneless, skinless chicken breasts
- 2 tablespoons fresh lime juice
- 1 tablespoon extra-virgin olive oil
- 1 tablespoon reduced-sodium soy sauce
- 1 tablespoon minced peeled fresh ginger
- 6 ounces sugar snap peas, strings removed

- Salt and freshly ground black pepper
- 1 medium ripe mango, peeled, pitted, and diced
- ½ medium cucumber, peeled, halved lengthwise, seeded, and diced
- ¼ cup chopped fresh mint leaves
- 3 ounces baby arugula leaves (about 4 handfuls)

In a large skillet, combine the chicken and lightly salted water to cover. Bring to a boil over high heat. Reduce the heat and simmer until cooked through but still juicy, about 12 minutes. Transfer to a cutting board and let cool slightly.

While the chicken is cooking, in a small bowl, whisk together the lime juice, oil, soy sauce, and ginger. Bring a small saucepan of salted water to a boil. Add the snap peas and cook for 30 seconds. Drain in a colander and rinse under cold running water. Drain again.

When the chicken is cool enough to handle, dice and transfer to a medium bowl. Add 2½ tablespoons of the dressing and toss. Season with salt and pepper to taste.

In a large bowl, toss the snap peas, mango, cucumber, mint, and arugula with the remaining dressing. Divide the snap pea mixture among 4 plates and top with the chicken.

NUTRITION AT A GLANCE
Per serving: 239 calories, 5 g fat, 1 g saturated fat, 32 g protein, 15 g carbohydrate, 3 g fiber, 247 mg sodium

Curried Turkey Salad

MAKES 4 servings   HANDS-ON TIME: 15 minutes   TOTAL TIME: 15 minutes

15
MINUTE
RECIPE

This supersimple version of a classic turkey salad uses deli turkey and a dressing lightened with yogurt. Seedless green grapes add sweetness.

⅓ cup nonfat plain yogurt

¼ cup mayonnaise

2 tablespoons fresh lime juice

2 teaspoons curry powder

¼ teaspoon ground ginger

    Salt and freshly ground black pepper

¾ pound lower-sodium deli roast turkey breast (½ inch thick), cut into ½-inch dice

¾ cup seedless green grapes, halved

1 celery stalk, cut into ¼-inch dice

3 tablespoons minced red onion

2 tablespoons minced fresh parsley

4 (8-inch) whole-wheat tortillas

4 large Bibb lettuce leaves

In a medium bowl, combine the yogurt, mayonnaise, lime juice, curry powder, ginger, and salt and pepper to taste. Add the turkey, grapes, celery, onion, and parsley and stir to combine.

Line the tortillas with the lettuce leaves and spoon about 1 cup turkey salad onto center of each. Fold the tortillas in half to serve.

NUTRITION AT A GLANCE

Per serving: 281 calories, 12 g fat, 2 g saturated fat, 20 g protein, 29 g carbohydrate, 3 g fiber, 794 mg sodium

Variation: For Phase 1, eliminate the grapes and tortillas and serve the salad on a bed of lettuce leaves.

Per serving (without grapes and tortilla): 189 calories, 11 g fat, 1.5 g saturated fat, 16 g protein, 4 g carbohydrate, 1 g fiber, 622 mg sodium

TIP: Keep in mind that curry powder is a blend of many spices and that no two blends are alike. You may wish to adjust the amount of curry powder you add to suit your taste.

Jalapeño Shrimp Salad

MAKES 4 (1½-cup) servings   HANDS-ON TIME: 10 minutes   TOTAL TIME: 15 minutes

Jalapeño pepper sauce is less vinegary than regular red hot sauce, which is why we use it here. Adding a little cayenne gives the marinade an extra boost of heat. You can substitute shredded red cabbage or a crisp lettuce like romaine for the endive if you prefer.

2	tablespoons jalapeño pepper sauce	4	teaspoons extra-virgin olive oil
2½	teaspoons dried oregano	1½	teaspoons Dijon mustard
½	teaspoon cayenne pepper	1	medium yellow squash
¼	teaspoon salt	1	medium zucchini
1½	pounds peeled and deveined extra-large shrimp	1	large Belgian endive (8 ounces), halved lengthwise and sliced crosswise into ½-inch-wide pieces
2	tablespoons red wine vinegar		

Heat a grill pan to medium. Or heat the broiler with the rack 4 inches from the heat.

In a large bowl, stir together the pepper sauce, 2 teaspoons of the oregano, the cayenne, and salt. Add the shrimp, tossing to coat well.

Grill or broil the shrimp for about 4 minutes, turning once during cooking, until pink and just opaque in the center.

Meanwhile, in a large bowl, whisk together the vinegar, oil, mustard, and remaining ½ teaspoon oregano. With a vegetable peeler, cut the yellow squash and zucchini into wide ribbons. Add to the dressing along with the endive and toss to coat.

Add the shrimp to the salad and toss. Divide the salad among 4 plates and serve.

NUTRITION AT A GLANCE
Per serving: 253 calories, 8 g fat, 1 g saturated fat, 36 g protein, 8 g carbohydrate, 3 g fiber, 636 mg sodium

TIP: Purchase endive that's wrapped in paper (it will have fewer brown spots from exposure to the light). Store in the cool part of the fridge.

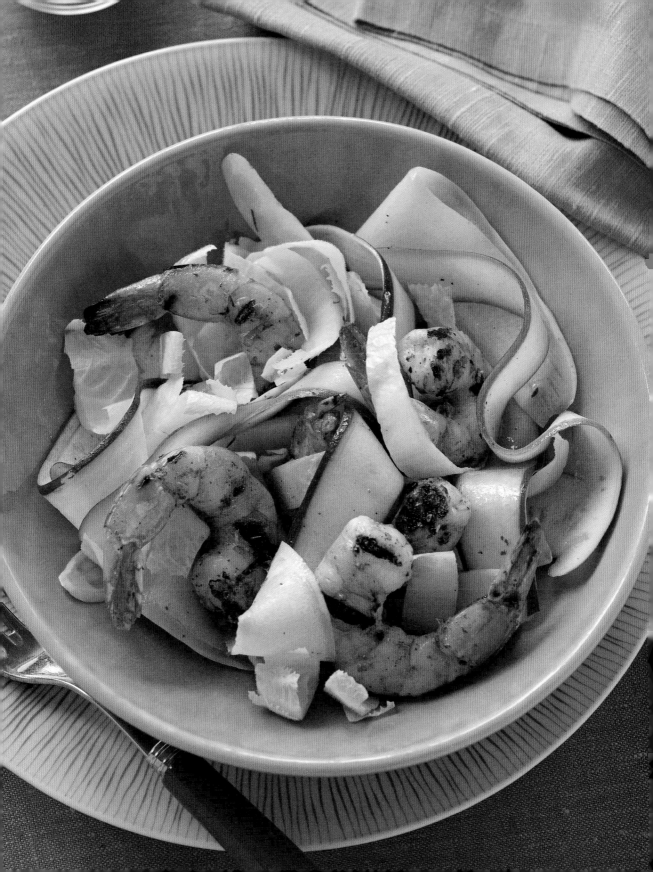

Pesto Pasta Salad

MAKES 4 servings   HANDS-ON TIME: 15 minutes   TOTAL TIME: 30 minutes

Adding spinach to already-healthy pesto keeps its color a brilliant green and boosts its vitamin and mineral power.

3 tablespoons pine nuts	1 tablespoon extra-virgin olive oil
1 medium garlic clove, unpeeled	⅓ cup grated Parmesan cheese
6 ounces whole-wheat penne	¼ cup fat-free cottage cheese
1½ cups packed fresh basil leaves	Salt and freshly ground black pepper
1 cup packed baby spinach leaves	2 medium tomatoes, coarsely chopped
1 tablespoon fresh lemon juice	

Bring a large pot of lightly salted water to a boil.

Meanwhile, in a small ungreased skillet over medium-low heat, toast the pine nuts, shaking the pan often, until golden and fragrant, 1 to 2 minutes. Pour onto a plate to stop the cooking.

Add the garlic to the boiling water and cook for 1 minute. Using a slotted spoon, remove from the water. When cool, peel and coarsely chop.

While the garlic is cooling, add the pasta to the boiling water and cook according to package directions. Reserving ¼ cup of the cooking water, drain the pasta in a colander and rinse under cool running water. Drain well.

While the pasta is cooking, make the pesto: In a food processor, pulse the pine nuts, garlic, basil, spinach, lemon juice, oil, and 2 tablespoons water until combined. Add the Parmesan and cottage cheese. Process until well combined. Season with salt and pepper to taste.

In a large serving bowl, toss the cooled pasta with the pesto, slowly adding reserved cooking water until the sauce is desired consistency. Fold in the tomatoes and serve.

NUTRITION AT A GLANCE
Per serving: 291 calories, 11 g fat, 2 g saturated fat, 12 g protein, 38 g carbohydrate, 5 g fiber, 177 mg sodium

Cook Once, Eat Twice

Double the recipe and add chunks of cooked chicken or pork to leftovers for a higher protein meal. Or make a double or triple batch of just the pesto and toss with steamed vegetables, such as broccoli, green beans, or carrots.

Quick Cobb Salad

MAKES 4 (2½-cup) servings   HANDS-ON TIME: 15 minutes   TOTAL TIME: 15 minutes

15 MINUTE RECIPE

If you can, buy the ham from the deli in one thick slice. If you can only get thin presliced ham, cut it into slivers instead of dice.

- ¼ cup extra-virgin olive oil
- 3 tablespoons fresh lemon juice
- ¼ teaspoon coarse sea salt
- ¼ teaspoon freshly ground black pepper
- 2 small heads romaine lettuce, shredded (about 8 cups)
- 1 cup no-salt-added canned black beans, drained and rinsed
- 6 ounces lower-sodium lean smoked ham, diced
- ¾ cup shredded part-skim mozzarella cheese (3 ounces)
- ½ avocado, diced

In a small bowl, whisk together the oil, lemon juice, salt, and pepper.

Place the lettuce in a large salad bowl and arrange rows of the beans, ham, mozzarella, and avocado on top.

Bring the salad to the table with the dressing on the side. Drizzle the dressing over the salad and toss.

NUTRITION AT A GLANCE
Per serving: 323 calories, 21 g fat, 5 g saturated fat, 18 g protein, 17 g carbohydrate, 6 g fiber, 596 mg sodium

Herbed Chicken and Bean Salad with Ranch Dressing

MAKES 4 (2-cup) servings   HANDS-ON TIME: 10 minutes   TOTAL TIME: 20 minutes

Poultry seasoning is a mix of many dried herbs, with sage and rosemary predominant. In this robust salad, it flavors the chicken and also sparks the homemade ranch dressing.

1½ teaspoons poultry seasoning	⅔ cup light (1.5%) buttermilk
¼ teaspoon salt	1 tablespoon mayonnaise
1 tablespoon extra-virgin olive oil	2 scallions, thinly sliced
1 pound boneless, skinless chicken breasts	1 can (15.5 ounces) small white beans, drained and rinsed
8 ounces green beans	
¼ teaspoon freshly ground black pepper	

Heat the oven to 450°F. Rub 1 teaspoon of the poultry seasoning, the salt, and oil onto both sides of the chicken breasts. Place the chicken in a shallow roasting pan and roast for 15 minutes, or until cooked through and still moist.

Meanwhile, in a shallow pan of simmering water, cook the green beans until crisp-tender, about 5 minutes. Drain, run under cold water to stop the cooking, and drain again.

In a large bowl, combine the remaining ½ teaspoon poultry seasoning and the pepper. Whisk in the buttermilk, mayonnaise, and scallions. Add the green beans and white beans and toss to coat.

Thinly slice the chicken crosswise, add to the bowl with the bean mixture, and toss to combine. Serve at room temperature.

NUTRITION AT A GLANCE
Per serving: 276 calories, 9 g fat, 2 g saturated fat, 34 g protein, 19 g carbohydrate, 6 g fiber, 559 mg sodium

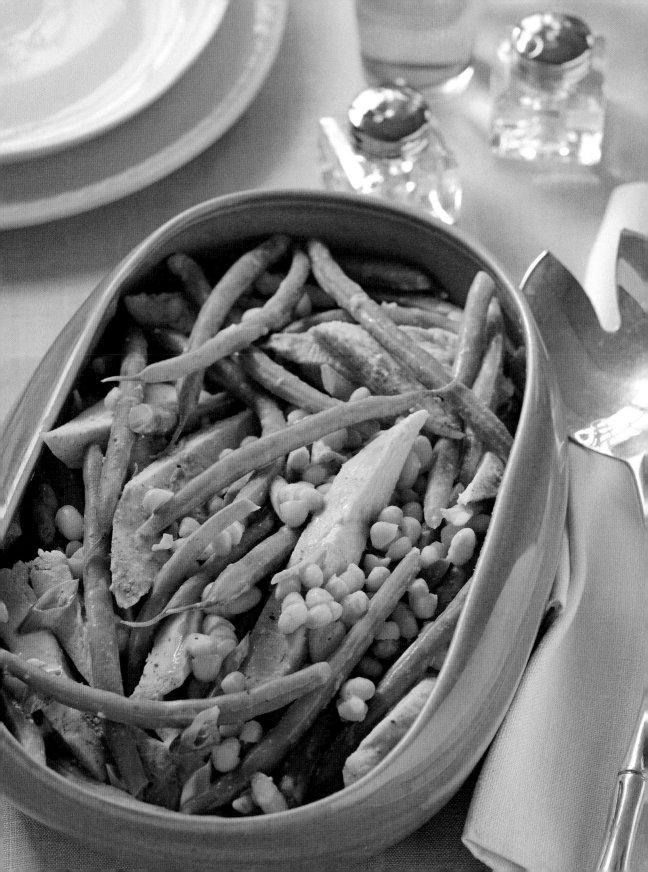

Warm Farro Salad

MAKES 4 (1½-cup) servings   HANDS-ON TIME: 15 minutes   TOTAL TIME: 20 minutes

An ancient Tuscan grain, farro is a healthy alternative to highly processed white rice. Its chewy texture and nutty flavor make it an ideal companion to black beans in this high-fiber salad.

1 cup semipearled farro

Salt

2 teaspoons extra-virgin olive oil

1 medium onion, chopped

1 medium zucchini, halved lengthwise and thinly sliced

1 can (10.5 ounces) black beans, drained and rinsed

Freshly ground black pepper

1 jar (6 ounces) roasted red peppers, drained and rinsed

¼ cup nonfat or low-fat plain yogurt

3 tablespoons fresh lime juice

1 teaspoon dark sesame oil

⅓ cup fresh basil leaves, slivered

In a medium-size heavy saucepan, combine the farro, 2½ cups water, and salt to taste. Bring to a boil over high heat. Reduce to a simmer and cook, uncovered, until just tender-chewy, about 15 minutes. Drain and transfer to a large serving bowl.

While the farro is cooking, in a large skillet, heat the olive oil over medium heat. Add the onion and zucchini and cook, stirring, until softened, about 5 minutes. Stir in the beans and cook just to warm through. Season with salt and black pepper to taste.

In a mini food processor or blender, combine half of the roasted peppers, the yogurt, lime juice, sesame oil, and black pepper to taste. Blend the dressing to a smooth purée.

Cut the remaining roasted peppers into slivers. Add the slivered peppers and the bean mixture to the bowl with the farro and toss well. Stir in the dressing, basil, and salt to taste. Serve warm or at room temperature.

NUTRITION AT A GLANCE
Per serving: 264 calories, 4 g fat, 0.5 g saturated fat, 12 g protein, 48 g carbohydrate, 7 g fiber, 288 mg sodium

TIP: Be sure to buy semipearled farro, which cooks in half the time of regular farro. Look for it in specialty food stores and Italian markets. If it's unavailable, you can use wheat berries instead (which will take longer to cook).

Chicken Salad Niçoise

MAKES 4 servings   HANDS-ON TIME: 25 minutes   TOTAL TIME: 25 minutes

Our Phase 1 rendition of the traditional French Niçoise salad uses economical chicken breast cutlets instead of tuna and eliminates the starchy white potatoes. To save time, buy a bag of already torn romaine.

- 1 pound thin-sliced chicken breast cutlets
- 2 teaspoons plus 3 tablespoons extra-virgin olive oil
- ¾ teaspoon dried oregano
-   Salt and black pepper
- ½ pound green beans, trimmed
- 3 tablespoons fresh lemon juice
- 1 tablespoon Dijon mustard
- 8 cups shredded or torn romaine lettuce (about 10 ounces)
- 2 large plum tomatoes, cut into thin wedges
- 16 pitted kalamata olives

Heat the broiler with the rack 6 inches from the heat.

In a medium bowl, toss the chicken with 2 teaspoons of the oil. Sprinkle both sides with the oregano and season lightly with salt and pepper. Place the chicken on a broiler pan and broil for 5 minutes, or until cooked through but still juicy. When cool enough to handle, cut the chicken crosswise into strips.

Meanwhile, in a steamer, cook the green beans for 3 to 5 minutes, until crisp-tender. Rinse under cold water to stop the cooking and drain well. In a small bowl, whisk together the remaining 3 tablespoons oil, the lemon juice, and mustard.

In a large bowl, toss the lettuce with 3 tablespoons of the dressing. Make a bed of lettuce on each of 4 serving plates. Top each with one-fourth of the chicken, green beans, tomatoes, and olives. Drizzle each salad with 1 tablespoon of the remaining dressing.

NUTRITION AT A GLANCE

Per serving: 284 calories, 15 g fat, 2 g saturated fat, 28 g protein, 9 g carbohydrate, 4 g fiber, 325 mg sodium

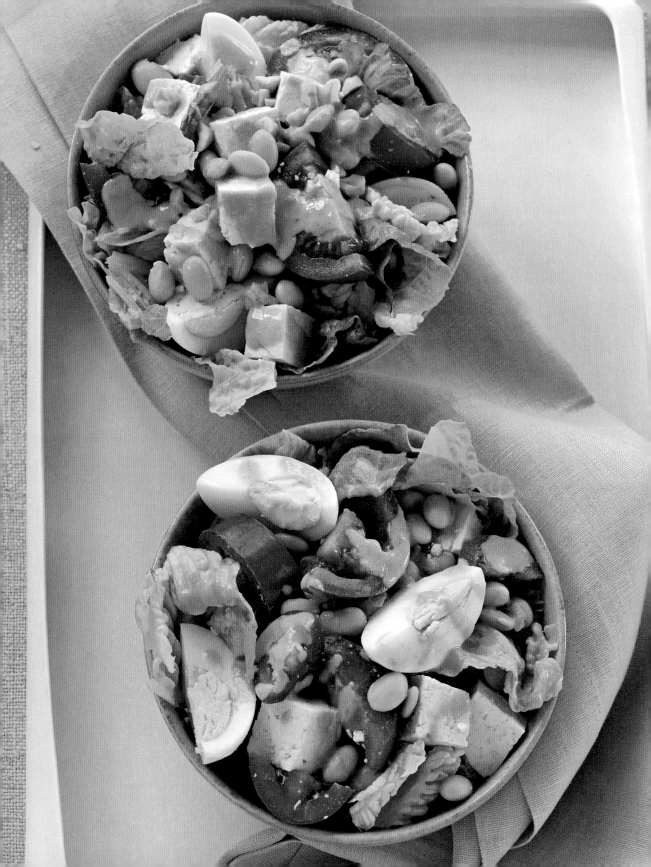

Double-Soy Salad

MAKES 4 (1¾-cup) servings   HANDS-ON TIME: 15 minutes   TOTAL TIME: 20 minutes

Fresh soybeans (edamame) and tofu provide plenty of soy protein in this pretty salad. The dressing calls for agave nectar (also called agave syrup), a sweetener you might not have used before. It's made from the juice of the Mexican agave cactus and is now available in many supermarkets in both light and dark versions.

- 3 large eggs
- 1½ cups frozen shelled edamame
- 4 teaspoons no-sugar-added creamy natural peanut butter
- 2 tablespoons rice vinegar
- ¾ teaspoon salt
- ½ teaspoon light agave nectar or ¼ teaspoon granular sugar substitute

- 12 ounces medium-firm tofu, cut into ½-inch chunks
- 4 plum tomatoes, halved lengthwise and sliced ½ inch thick
- 3 cups shredded romaine lettuce (4 ounces)
- 10 dry-roasted raw peanuts, chopped

Place the eggs in a small saucepan with cold water to cover. Bring to a boil over high heat. Remove from the heat, cover, and let stand for 12 minutes. Run the eggs under cold water and drain. Peel and quarter lengthwise.

While the eggs sit, in a small saucepan of boiling water, cook the edamame until tender, 3 minutes. Drain, run under cold water, and drain again.

In a large bowl, whisk together the peanut butter, vinegar, salt, agave nectar, and 2 tablespoons water until smooth. Add the hard-boiled eggs, edamame, tofu, tomatoes, and romaine. Toss to combine.

Divide the salad among 4 plates and sprinkle each with chopped peanuts.

NUTRITION AT A GLANCE
Per serving: 268 calories, 14 g fat, 2 g saturated fat, 21 g protein, 15 g carbohydrate, 6 g fiber, 541 mg sodium

Speedy Fajita Salad

MAKES 4 servings   HANDS-ON TIME: 20 minutes   TOTAL TIME: 20 minutes

This Mexican favorite, transformed into a Phase 1 lunch or dinner salad, is a boon for busy days because it calls for lean deli roast beef. Look for packaged taco seasoning (typically a mixture of garlic, oregano, cumin, and chili powder) in the Mexican section of the grocery.

¾ pound thinly sliced lower-sodium lean deli roast beef

1 tablespoon prepared taco seasoning

3 teaspoons extra-virgin olive oil

½ large red bell pepper, thinly sliced

½ large yellow or green bell pepper, thinly sliced

4 cups chopped romaine lettuce

1 cup chopped tomato

½ cup diced red onion

3 tablespoons fresh lime juice

¼ cup shredded reduced-fat Monterey Jack cheese (1 ounce)

¼ cup chopped fresh cilantro or parsley

In a medium bowl, combine the beef and taco seasoning, tossing to coat.

In a large nonstick skillet, heat 1 teaspoon of the oil over medium-low heat. Add the bell peppers and cook, stirring often, until softened, about 4 minutes. Add the beef and cook, stirring occasionally, just to heat through, about 2 minutes.

Meanwhile, place the lettuce, tomato, and onion in a large serving bowl. In a cup, whisk together the lime juice and remaining 2 teaspoons oil. Pour over the lettuce mixture and toss to coat.

Divide the lettuce mixture among 4 plates and top with the beef and peppers. Sprinkle evenly with the cheese and cilantro and serve warm.

NUTRITION AT A GLANCE
Per serving: 216 calories, 9 g fat, 3 g saturated fat, 26 g protein, 11 g carbohydrate, 2 g fiber, 400 mg sodium

Variation: For Phase 2, serve the beef mixture with warmed whole-wheat tortillas and the lettuce mixture.
Per serving (with tortilla): 346 calories, 11 g fat, 3 g saturated fat, 30 g protein, 37 g carbohydrate, 5 g fiber, 730 mg sodium

Chunky Gazpacho Salad with Grilled Scallops

MAKES 4 servings   **HANDS-ON TIME:** 15 minutes   **TOTAL TIME:** 15 minutes

Grilled scallops provide protein in this summer salad, which is reminiscent of the classic gazpacho (a chilled cucumber–tomato soup), but you could substitute grilled shrimp. Lightly coat the grill with a little oil so the seafood doesn't stick. Not a fan of raw garlic? Just leave it out or blanch it for a few minutes before mashing.

2 garlic cloves, minced

½ teaspoon salt, plus additional to taste

4 medium tomatoes, seeded and diced

1 medium cucumber, peeled, halved lengthwise, seeded, and diced

1 large red bell pepper, diced

1 small onion, minced

3 tablespoons sherry vinegar

1 tablespoon extra-virgin olive oil

Freshly ground black pepper

1¼ pounds sea scallops

1 large lime, quartered, for serving

Heat the broiler. Or heat a grill to medium–high.

On a cutting board, using a fork, mash the garlic with ½ teaspoon salt until pasty. Scrape into a large mixing bowl. Add the tomatoes, cucumber, bell pepper, onion, vinegar, and oil and toss to combine. Let stand for 5 minutes to allow the vegetables to give off their juices. Season to taste with salt and pepper.

Meanwhile, pat the scallops dry and season lightly with salt. Broil or grill for 2 minutes per side, or until lightly browned on the outsides and just opaque in the centers.

Divide the gazpacho salad among 4 shallow bowls. Top with the scallops. Serve with lime wedges for squeezing.

NUTRITION AT A GLANCE
Per serving: 214 calories, 5 g fat, 0.5 g saturated fat, 26 g protein, 16 g carbohydrate, 3 g fiber, 530 mg sodium

TIP: This salad is delicious at the height of summer when you can use beefsteak tomatoes at their best. Beefsteaks are juicier and easier to chop than plum tomatoes (which you can use at other times of year).

Asian Roast Pork Salad

MAKES 4 (1½-cup) servings HANDS-ON TIME: 10 minutes TOTAL TIME: 30 minutes

Look for Asian pears in supermarkets from July through September. The round fruit, with yellow-green to russet skin, is crunchy like an apple but tastes more like a mild pear. If you can't find an Asian pear, use a Bosc pear instead.

- 3 tablespoons balsamic vinegar
- 1½ teaspoons garam masala
- ½ teaspoon ground ginger
- ½ teaspoon salt
- ¼ teaspoon freshly ground black pepper
- 1 (¾-pound) pork tenderloin, well trimmed

- 4 teaspoons extra-virgin olive oil
- 2 Kirby cucumbers, peeled in stripes and thinly sliced
- 2 celery stalks, thinly sliced
- 1 Asian pear (about 10 ounces), cored and thinly sliced

Heat the oven to 450°F. Line a rimmed baking sheet with foil.

In a small bowl, stir together 1 tablespoon of the vinegar, 1 teaspoon of the garam masala, the ginger, salt, and pepper. Place the pork on the baking sheet and brush with the vinegar mixture. Roast for about 20 minutes, until an instant-read thermometer inserted into the center registers 155°F and the juices run clear. Let the pork sit for 5 minutes.

While the pork is roasting, in a large bowl, whisk together the remaining 2 tablespoons vinegar, remaining ½ teaspoon garam masala, and the oil. Add the cucumbers, celery, and pear and toss to combine.

Thinly slice the pork. Add to bowl and toss to combine. Serve the salad warm or at room temperature.

NUTRITION AT A GLANCE
Per serving: 197 calories, 8 g fat, 2 g saturated fat, 20 g protein, 13 g carbohydrate, 4 g fiber, 360 mg sodium

TIP: Look for garam masala in Indian markets or your supermarket. There are many variations of this Indian spice mix, which typically contains cinnamon, cloves, coriander, cardamom, cumin, and sometimes dried chiles in hotter versions. Experiment to find a mix you like best.

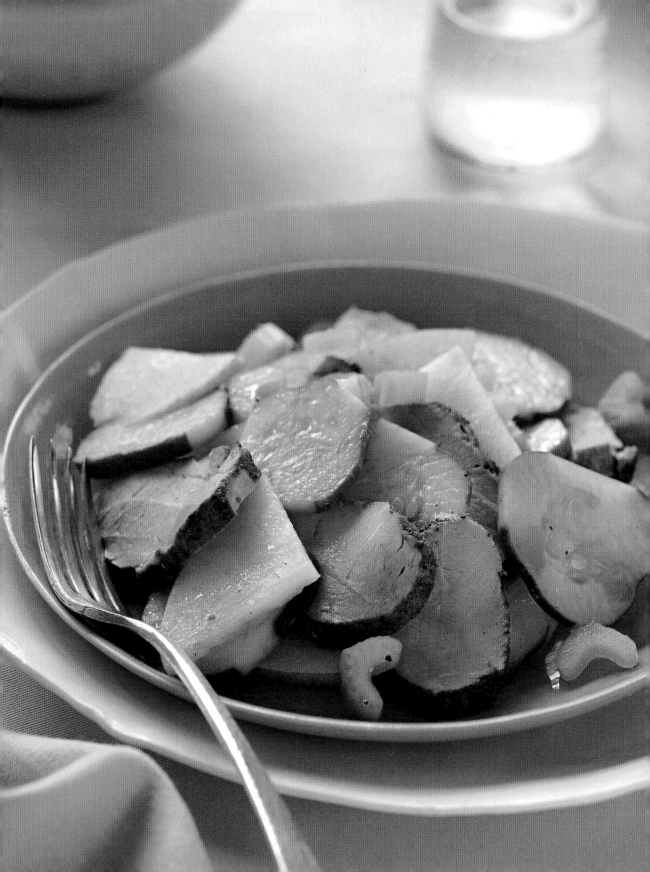

Buffalo Chicken Salad

MAKES 4 (1⅓-cup) servings   HANDS-ON TIME: 15 minutes   TOTAL TIME: 25 minutes

If you crave buffalo chicken wings, you'll enjoy the similar flavors (including the blue cheese dressing) in this healthy salad. To save time, cut up the vegetables while the chicken is cooking.

- 3 garlic cloves, smashed and peeled
- 1 teaspoon red pepper flakes
- ½ teaspoon salt
- 1½ pounds boneless, skinless chicken breasts
- ⅓ cup light (1.5%) buttermilk
- ½ cup crumbled reduced-fat blue cheese (2 ounces)
- 1 teaspoon extra-virgin olive oil
- 1 teaspoon hot pepper sauce
- 2 celery stalks, diced
- 1 medium red bell pepper, diced
- 1 package (5 ounces) mixed field greens

In a 10- or 12-inch skillet, combine the garlic, red pepper flakes, salt, and 1 inch of water (about 3 cups). Bring to a high simmer over high heat.

Meanwhile, cut the chicken crosswise into 1-inch-wide strips.

Add the chicken to the cooking liquid, cover, and simmer over medium-low heat for 5 minutes. Remove the pan from the heat and let sit for 5 minutes.

Meanwhile, in a mini food processor or blender, combine the buttermilk, blue cheese, oil, and hot pepper sauce. Process to a smooth purée.

Drain the chicken, discarding the broth, and spread out on a cutting board to cool slightly. In a medium bowl, combine the celery and bell pepper. Cut the chicken into bite-size pieces and add to the vegetables. Add the blue cheese dressing and toss well.

Line 4 plates with field greens and top with the chicken salad.

NUTRITION AT A GLANCE
Per serving: 272 calories, 7 g fat, 3 g saturated fat, 45 g protein, 6 g carbohydrate, 2 g fiber, 667 mg sodium

Spinach and Bean Salad with Shrimp

MAKES 4 servings   HANDS-ON TIME: 25 minutes   TOTAL TIME: 25 minutes

This satisfying main-course salad is elegant enough for company, yet comes together quickly for a weekday meal. If you make it ahead of time, wait until you're ready to serve it before dressing the greens.

1½ pounds peeled and deveined jumbo shrimp

2 teaspoons grated lemon zest

3 tablespoons fresh lemon juice

Salt and freshly ground black pepper

2 teaspoons plus 1 tablespoon extra-virgin olive oil

1 small red bell pepper, thinly sliced

1 pound asparagus, cut on the diagonal into 1-inch pieces

2 tablespoons minced shallot

¾ cup canned white beans, drained and rinsed

1 tablespoon chopped fresh tarragon leaves

1 bag (6 ounces) baby spinach leaves

Heat a grill pan to medium-high.

In a medium bowl, combine the shrimp, lemon zest, and 2 tablespoons of the lemon juice. Season lightly with salt and pepper. Set aside.

In a medium nonstick skillet, heat 2 teaspoons of the oil over medium heat. Add the bell pepper and cook, stirring occasionally, for 2 minutes. Add the asparagus and cook, stirring occasionally, for 2 minutes. Add the shallot and cook, stirring, for 1 minute longer. Transfer the vegetables to a large bowl, add the beans, and set aside.

Lightly coat the grill pan with a little oil. Cook the shrimp for about 2 minutes per side, until they turn pink and just opaque in the center. Transfer to a plate.

In a cup, whisk together the remaining 1 tablespoon lemon juice, remaining 1 tablespoon oil, and tarragon. Add salt and pepper to taste.

Add the spinach and dressing to the vegetable and bean mixture and toss to coat.

Divide the salad among 4 plates and top with the grilled shrimp.

NUTRITION AT A GLANCE
Per serving: 316 calories, 9 g fat, 1 g saturated fat, 41 g protein, 21 g carbohydrate, 7 g fiber, 488 mg sodium

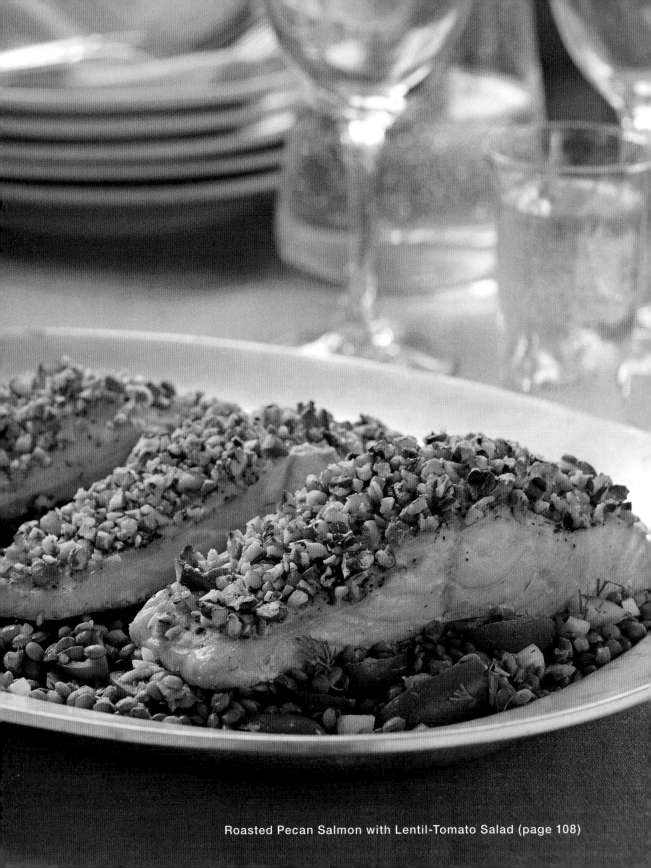

Roasted Pecan Salmon with Lentil-Tomato Salad (page 108)

FISH AND SHELLFISH

When it comes to quick and healthy cooking, fish and shellfish should be on your menu at least twice a week, both for their healthful nutrients and for their ease of preparation. Whether you choose to bake the mackerel, sauté the shrimp, oven "fry" the fish sticks, pan-sear the cod, or roast the salmon, you can have almost any type of seafood on the table in minutes. Moreover, fatty fish like salmon and mackerel supply heart-healthy omega-3 fatty acids along with bone-strengthening vitamin D, while leaner fish like sole, cod, and snapper are good sources of B vitamins. And don't worry about shrimp; they won't raise your cholesterol.

Always choose the freshest seafood you can find and avoid fish that are high in mercury and other contaminants, such as swordfish, king mackerel, and tilefish. And remember that seafood freezes well for a few weeks. Look for great buys on salmon and fresh tuna and stock up for future meals.

Roasted Pecan Salmon with Lentil-Tomato Salad

MAKES 4 servings   HANDS-ON TIME: 20 minutes   TOTAL TIME: 30 minutes

This fish entrée is so elegant no one will ever suspect you made it in half an hour. We recommend using flavorful French Le Puy lentils, which cook in 20 minutes and keep their shape beautifully. You could use 1 cup of drained and rinsed canned lentils, if you prefer.

½ cup dried small green Le Puy lentils

4 (6-ounce) salmon fillets, with skin

Salt and freshly ground black pepper

4 teaspoons Dijon mustard

½ cup chopped pecan halves

½ cup halved cherry or grape tomatoes

1 large shallot, minced

1 tablespoon chopped fresh dill

1 tablespoon fresh lemon juice

1 tablespoon extra-virgin olive oil

1 teaspoon red wine vinegar

Heat the oven to 425°F. Lightly coat a baking sheet with cooking spray.

In a medium saucepan, bring the lentils and 2 cups of water to a boil. Reduce the heat to a simmer and cook, uncovered, until the lentils are just tender but not mushy, 15 to 20 minutes.

While the lentils are cooking, place the salmon on the baking sheet and season with salt and pepper. Spread each fillet with 1 teaspoon of the mustard, then top each with 2 tablespoons chopped pecans. Roast the salmon for 10 to 12 minutes, until the fish just flakes when tested with a fork.

Meanwhile, make the salad: In a medium bowl, combine the tomatoes, shallot, dill, lemon juice, oil, and vinegar. Add the lentils and salt and pepper to taste. Toss well.

Divide the salad among 4 plates and top with the salmon.

NUTRITION AT A GLANCE
Per serving (with ½ cup salad): 522 calories, 32 g fat, 5 g saturated fat, 41 g protein, 18 g carbohydrate, 5 g fiber, 229 mg sodium

Striped Bass Roasted with Cauliflower, Lemon, and Olives

MAKES 4 servings   HANDS-ON TIME: 10 minutes   TOTAL TIME: 30 minutes

A white-on-white main course makes refined party fare and this recipe is easily doubled for a crowd. Use the best olives you can find; kalamata or green Spanish olives would be delicious here.

1   large lemon

2   cups small cauliflower florets

8   pitted black or green olives, halved

3   garlic cloves, thinly sliced

2   tablespoons extra-virgin olive oil

4   (6-ounce) skinless striped bass fillets

½   teaspoon dried oregano

½   teaspoon salt

Heat the oven to 450°F.

With a small sharp knife, cut a slice off the top and bottom of the lemon. Following the curve of the fruit, remove the zest and white pith. Dice the lemon flesh, discarding the seeds.

In a 9 × 13-inch baking pan, toss the diced lemon, cauliflower, olives, and garlic with 1 tablespoon of the oil. Push the mixture to all 4 sides of pan.

Place the fish in 1 layer in the center of the pan and season with the oregano and salt. Drizzle the remaining 1 tablespoon oil over the fish. Roast for 20 minutes, or until the fish is just cooked through and flakes when tested with a fork.

Transfer the fish and cauliflower mixture to 4 plates. Serve hot.

NUTRITION AT A GLANCE
Per serving: 265 calories, 12 g fat, 2 g saturated fat, 31 g protein, 5 g carbohydrate, 2 g fiber, 511 mg sodium

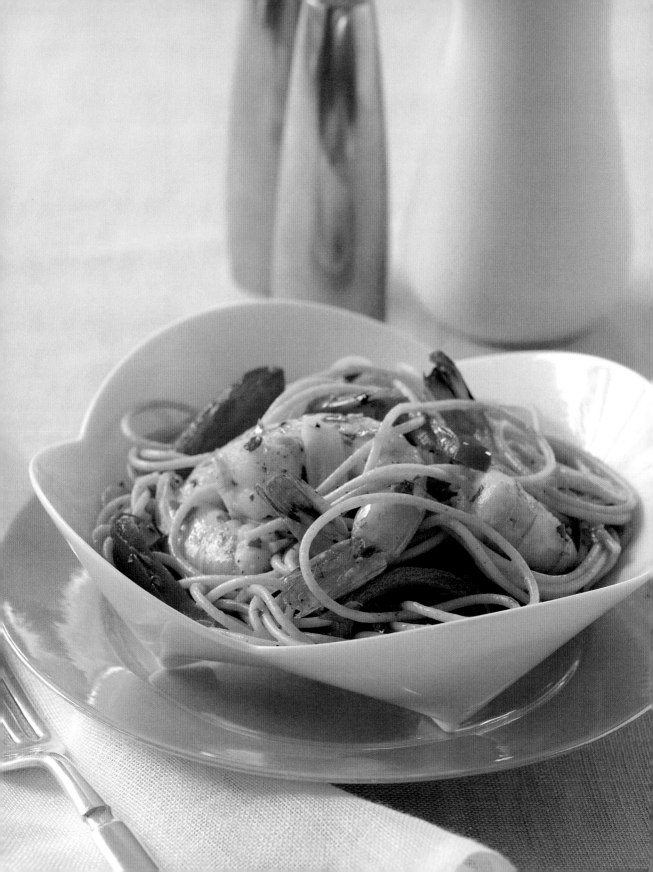

Shrimp Scampi with Whole-Wheat Pasta

MAKES 4 servings   HANDS-ON TIME: 15 minutes   TOTAL TIME: 25 minutes

We've improved this quick classic by replacing the usual butter with monounsaturated extra-virgin olive oil. And we've switched out highly processed white pasta for high-fiber whole-wheat. (For a Phase 1 version, see the Variation.) Using peeled and deveined shrimp makes preparing the dish a breeze.

8 ounces whole-wheat spaghetti or cappellini

3 tablespoons extra-virgin olive oil

1 medium red bell pepper, thinly sliced

5 large garlic cloves, minced

½ cup white wine or lower-sodium chicken broth

⅛ teaspoon red pepper flakes, or to taste

1½ pounds peeled and deveined large shrimp

2 tablespoons fresh lemon juice

⅓ cup chopped fresh parsley

Salt and freshly ground black pepper

Bring a large pot of lightly salted water to a boil. Add the pasta and cook according to package directions. Drain.

While the pasta is cooking, in large nonstick skillet, heat the oil over medium-high heat. Add the bell pepper and cook, stirring, for 2 minutes. Add the garlic and cook, stirring, for 1 minute. Add the wine and pepper flakes. Bring to a simmer and cook until the liquid is slightly reduced, about 1 minute longer.

Add the shrimp and cook, stirring, until they turn pink and are just opaque in the center, about 3 minutes. Remove the pan from the heat and stir in the lemon juice.

In a large serving bowl, combine the drained pasta, shrimp mixture, and parsley. Season with salt and pepper to taste. Toss well and serve.

NUTRITION AT A GLANCE
Per serving: 490 calories, 14 g fat, 2 g saturated fat, 44 g protein, 48 g carbohydrate, 8 g fiber, 261 mg sodium

Variation: If you're on Phase 1, simply serve the shrimp on 1 cup of sautéed baby spinach and omit the pasta.
Per serving (with spinach instead of pasta): 315 calories, 14 g fat, 2 g saturated fat, 38 g protein, 10 g carbohydrate, 4 g fiber, 449 mg sodium

15 MINUTE RECIPE

Sole à la Meunière

MAKES 4 servings   HANDS-ON TIME: 5 minutes   TOTAL TIME: 10 minutes

The French word *meunière* means "miller's wife" and refers to a rustic style of cooking in which fish fillets are dredged in flour and then browned in butter. In this healthier take on the classic, we use chickpea flour for coating the fish and olive oil for cooking it. The dish is then finished with a piquant sauce made from trans-fat-free margarine and capers. For information on chickpea flour, see page 67.

- ¼ cup chickpea flour
- 4 (6-ounce) sole fillets
- ½ teaspoon salt
- 4 teaspoons extra-virgin olive oil
- 3 tablespoons fresh lemon juice
- 2 teaspoons nonpareil capers, drained and rinsed
- 2 teaspoons cold trans-fat-free margarine (vegetable oil spread)
- ¼ cup whole parsley leaves

Place the chickpea flour in a pie plate or shallow bowl. Sprinkle the fillets with the salt. Dredge the fillets in the flour, shaking off excess.

In a large nonstick skillet, heat 2 teaspoons of the oil over medium-high heat. Add 2 fillets to the skillet and cook until crisp, browned, and cooked through, about 1 minute per side. Transfer to a platter and keep warm. Repeat with the remaining 2 teaspoons oil and remaining fish.

To the same skillet, add the lemon juice, capers, and 2 tablespoons water. Cook for 30 seconds, scraping up any browned bits that cling to the bottom of the pan. Remove the pan from the heat and swirl in the margarine.

Transfer a fillet to each of 4 plates, sprinkle with the parsley leaves, and spoon 1 tablespoon sauce over each.

NUTRITION AT A GLANCE
Per serving: 237 calories, 9 g fat, 2 g saturated fat, 34 g protein, 5 g carbohydrate, 1 g fiber, 492 mg sodium

TIP: If you can't find tiny nonpareil capers, coarsely chop larger capers for this recipe.

Pan-Seared Cod with Pine Nut Gremolata

MAKES 4 servings **HANDS-ON TIME: 20 minutes** **TOTAL TIME: 20 minutes**

Gremolata is a traditional Italian garnish of lemon zest, parsley, and garlic. We've added pine nuts for a flavorful and healthful twist (they're high in phytosterols). It's a sensational topping for mild-flavored cod.

- 4 (5-ounce) skinless cod fillets
- ½ teaspoon salt
- Freshly ground black pepper
- 1 lemon
- ¼ cup finely chopped fresh parsley
- 2 large garlic cloves, minced

- 2 tablespoons pine nuts, coarsely chopped
- 2 tablespoons extra-virgin olive oil
- 1 seedless cucumber (about 10 inches long), thinly sliced on the diagonal

Season the fillets with ¼ teaspoon of the salt and pepper to taste.

Grate 1 tablespoon zest from lemon. In a small bowl, combine the zest, parsley, garlic, pine nuts, and remaining ¼ teaspoon salt. Halve the lemon and set aside.

In a large nonstick skillet, heat the oil over medium-high heat. Add the fish and cook until lightly browned on 1 side, about 3 minutes. Carefully turn the fish over. Squeeze lemon juice over the fillets and cook for 4 minutes longer, or until the fish just flakes when tested with a fork.

Arrange the cucumber slices on 4 plates in an overlapping pattern. Lay the fillets over the cucumbers, top with the gremolata, and serve.

NUTRITION AT A GLANCE
Per serving: 223 calories, 11 g fat, 1 g saturated fat, 27 g protein, 4 g carbohydrate, 1 g fiber, 381 mg sodium

TIP: Flat white fish, like cod and flounder, cook in a flash and can therefore easily be overcooked. To ensure perfectly moist fillets, get your oiled pan hot before adding the fish.

Tilapia Margarita

MAKES 4 servings   HANDS-ON TIME: 10 minutes   TOTAL TIME: 20 minutes

This south-of-the-border-inspired dish is sparked with a little tequila. If you'd rather not use it, add an additional tablespoon of orange juice instead. Look for fresh, dark green, mildly hot poblano chiles in the produce aisle of your supermarket.

1 teaspoon salt	½ cup diced poblano chile
½ teaspoon ground allspice	1 scallion, thinly sliced
½ teaspoon freshly ground black pepper	½ cup fresh orange juice
4 (5- to 6-ounce) skinless tilapia fillets	2 tablespoons fresh lime juice
	1 tablespoon tequila
4 teaspoons extra-virgin olive oil	Lime wedges, for serving

In a small bowl, stir together the salt, allspice, and pepper. Season the fillets on both sides with the spice mixture.

In a large nonstick skillet, heat 1 teaspoon of the oil over medium heat. Add 2 fillets and cook until golden brown on the outside and the fish just flakes when tested with a fork, about 2 minutes per side. Transfer the fish to a platter. Repeat with 1 teaspoon of the remaining oil and the remaining fish.

Add the poblano and scallion to the pan and cook until the poblano is just tender, 1 minute. Remove the pan from the heat and add the orange juice, lime juice, and tequila. Return the pan to the heat and cook for 1 minute. Add the remaining 2 teaspoons oil, bring to a boil, and swirl to emulsify and thicken the sauce.

Spoon the sauce over the fish on the platter and serve hot with lime wedges for squeezing.

NUTRITION AT A GLANCE
Per serving: 206 calories, 7 g fat, 2 g saturated fat, 29 g protein, 6 g carbohydrate, 1 g fiber, 657 mg sodium

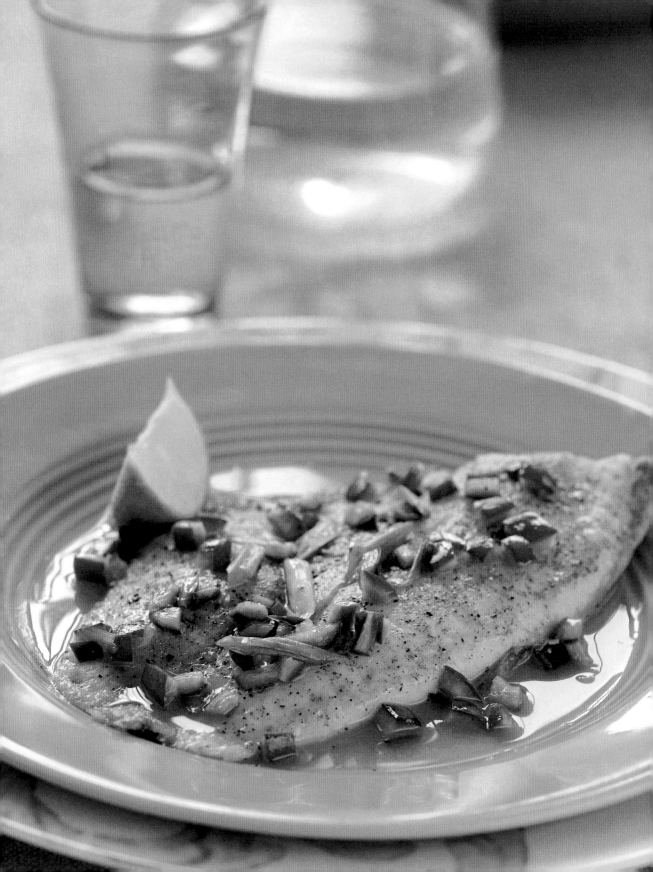

15
MINUTE
RECIPE

Seared Salmon in Creamy Dill Sauce

MAKES 4 servings   HANDS-ON TIME: 10 minutes   TOTAL TIME: 15 minutes

Salmon is a rich source of heart–healthy omega-3 fatty acids. We recommend intensely flavored wild salmon because it contains less mercury and other contaminants than farm-raised.

¼ cup low-fat mayonnaise

½ cup nonfat (0%) plain Greek yogurt

4 scallions, thinly sliced

¼ cup chopped fresh dill

3 tablespoons fresh lemon juice

4 (6-ounce) salmon fillets, with skin

Salt and freshly ground black pepper

1 tablespoon extra-virgin olive oil

2 ounces alfalfa sprouts (2 cups)

In a small bowl, combine the mayonnaise, yogurt, scallions, dill, and lemon juice. Season the salmon with salt and pepper.

In a large nonstick skillet, heat the oil over medium-high heat. Add the salmon, flesh-side down, and sear until browned, about 3 minutes. Turn and sear the skin side until the salmon just flakes when tested with a fork, about 3 minutes longer.

Spoon 3 tablespoons of the dill sauce onto each of 4 plates and top with a salmon fillet and a sprinkling of sprouts.

NUTRITION AT A GLANCE
Per serving: 419 calories, 27 g fat, 6 g saturated fat, 37 g protein, 5 g carbohydrate, 1 g fiber, 235 mg sodium

Garlic Shrimp
with Swiss Chard and Chickpeas

MAKES 4 servings   HANDS-ON TIME: 15 minutes   TOTAL TIME: 25 minutes

Nutrient-rich Swiss chard, a leafy green vegetable that resembles spinach, is a delicious addition to this seafood dish. Chard is an excellent source of vitamins A, C, and K and is also high in vitamin E. The chickpeas provide filling fiber.

1 tablespoon extra-virgin olive oil

1 medium bunch Swiss chard (about 12 ounces), trimmed and coarsely chopped

1 cup halved cherry tomatoes

2 scallions, thinly sliced

4 garlic cloves, minced

1½ pounds peeled and deveined large shrimp

1 cup no-salt-added canned chickpeas, drained and rinsed

Salt and freshly ground black pepper

¼ cup crumbled reduced-fat feta cheese (1 ounce)

In a large nonstick skillet, heat the oil over medium heat. Add the chard, tomatoes, scallions, and garlic. Cook, stirring occasionally, until the chard is wilted, about 5 minutes.

Add the shrimp and chickpeas and cook until the shrimp turn pink and are just opaque in the center, 3 to 5 minutes longer.

Spoon the shrimp mixture into 4 bowls and top each serving with 1 tablespoon feta.

NUTRITION AT A GLANCE
Per serving: 324 calories, 8 g fat, 2 g saturated fat, 42 g protein, 19 g carbohydrate, 5 g fiber, 569 mg sodium

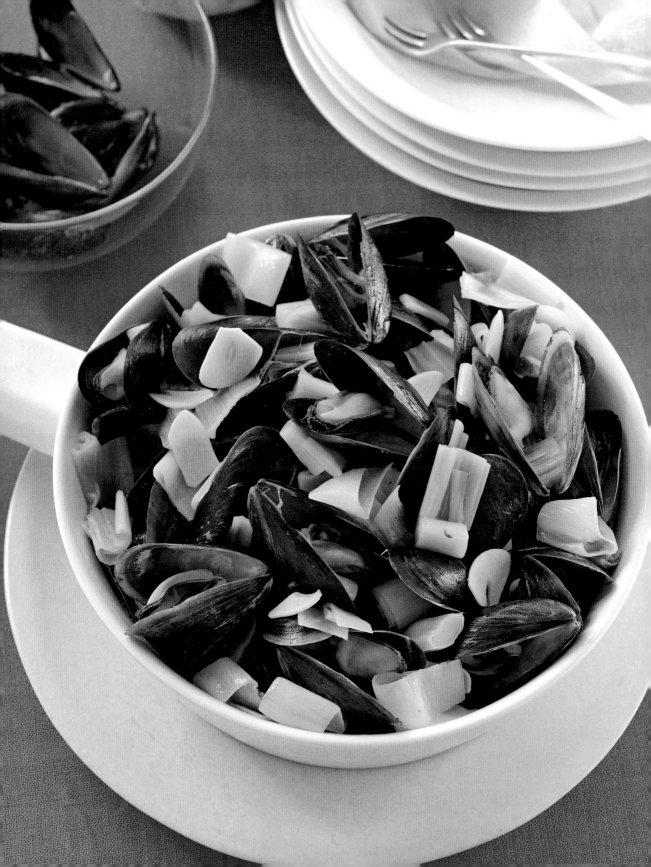

Mussels and Leeks in Fennel Broth

MAKES 4 servings   HANDS-ON TIME: 20 minutes   TOTAL TIME: 30 minutes

When you clean mussels, be sure to pull out any beards. Before steaming, discard any mussels with broken shells or those that don't close if you tap them on the counter. Because much of the wine evaporates, you can serve this as a Phase 1 dish. If you're on Phase 2, enjoy with a piece of a whole-wheat baguette for dipping into the broth.

4 teaspoons extra-virgin olive oil	4 medium leeks
2 garlic cloves, slivered	3 pounds mussels, debearded
½ teaspoon fennel seeds, lightly crushed	⅓ cup dry white wine

In a large heavy pot, heat the oil, garlic, and fennel seeds over low heat until fragrant, about 3 minutes.

Meanwhile, trim the root ends and all but 1 inch of the dark green tops from the leeks. Halve lengthwise, then cut crosswise into 1-inch slices. Place the sliced leeks in a large bowl of warm water and swish around to remove any sand or grit (which will fall to the bottom of the bowl). Carefully lift the leeks out of the water and drain well in a colander.

Add the leeks to the pot. Increase the heat to medium-high, and cook, stirring often, until the leeks begin to soften, about 5 minutes.

Add the mussels and wine. Cover tightly and steam for 8 minutes, until the mussels open (stir the mussels about halfway through to be sure they cook evenly). Discard any mussels that haven't opened by the end of the cooking time.

Spoon the mussels and leeks into 4 shallow bowls. Divide the broth evenly among the bowls and serve.

NUTRITION AT A GLANCE
Per serving: 373 calories, 12 g fat, 2 g saturated fat, 37 g protein, 25 g carbohydrate, 2 g fiber, 877 mg sodium

Baked Parmesan-Stuffed Mackerel

MAKES 4 servings   HANDS-ON TIME: 10 minutes   TOTAL TIME: 30 minutes

Mackerel is an oily fish that's a great source of heart-healthy omega-3 fatty acids and vitamin B_{12} (a 3-ounce serving provides nearly 700 percent of the RDA for B_{12}). Be sure to use the smaller Spanish mackerel and not king mackerel (which can be high in mercury). Or try very fresh bluefish instead.

1 package (10 ounces) frozen chopped spinach, thawed and squeezed dry

½ cup grated Parmesan cheese (2 ounces)

4 (6-ounce) skinless Spanish mackerel fillets

Salt

1 can (14.5 ounces) diced tomatoes with garlic, with juice

½ teaspoon dried oregano

3 strips orange zest

Heat the oven to 450°F.

In a medium bowl, stir together the spinach and Parmesan. Season the fillets on both sides with salt. Spread the spinach mixture over the flat side of each fillet. Fold the fillets in half crosswise.

In a 9 × 9-inch baking pan, stir together the tomatoes and their juice, oregano, and orange zest. Place the fillets in the pan and cover with foil. Bake for about 20 minutes, until the sauce is bubbly and the fish flakes when tested with a fork. Serve hot with the sauce.

NUTRITION AT A GLANCE
Per serving: 323 calories, 15 g fat, 6 g saturated fat, 41 g protein, 4 g carbohydrate, 2 g fiber, 413 mg sodium

Cod with Cabbage and Bacon

MAKES 4 servings   HANDS-ON TIME: 10 minutes   TOTAL TIME: 30 minutes

The skillet goes from the stovetop right into the oven for this one-dish meal that's so simple to make you'll want to prepare it time and again. Turkey bacon adds a smokiness to the mild cod and also flavors the cabbage. The broth keeps the fish moist during baking.

1 tablespoon extra-virgin olive oil

3 strips turkey bacon, chopped

½ head (12 ounces) napa cabbage, shredded (4 cups)

⅓ cup clam broth or lower-sodium chicken broth

1 teaspoon dried tarragon

4 (6-ounce) skinless cod fillets

½ teaspoon salt

¼ teaspoon freshly ground black pepper

Heat the oven to 425°F.

In a large ovenproof skillet, heat the oil over medium heat. Add the bacon and cook until lightly crisped, about 2 minutes. Add the cabbage and cook, stirring frequently, until wilted, about 5 minutes. Add the broth and tarragon and bring to a boil.

Place the cod on top of the cabbage and sprinkle with the salt and pepper. Cover the pan, place in the oven, and bake for about 15 minutes, until the fish flakes with a fork and the cabbage is tender. Serve hot.

NUTRITION AT A GLANCE
Per serving: 213 calories, 6 g fat, 1 g saturated fat, 36 g protein, 2 g carbohydrate, 1 g fiber, 436 mg sodium

TIP: Don't confuse Chinese napa cabbage with its relative, bok choy. Napa's leaves are crinkly and white to light green, while bok choy has white stems and dark green leaves.

Baked Halibut with Asparagus and Shiitake Mushrooms

MAKES 4 servings   HANDS-ON TIME: 10 minutes   TOTAL TIME: 25 minutes

This is a pretty dish that makes great company fare. You can substitute snapper if halibut isn't available. Be sure to remove and discard the shiitake stems; they can be very tough.

- 12 ounces asparagus, trimmed and cut into 2-inch lengths
- 8 ounces shiitake mushrooms, stems removed, caps halved if large
- 3 scallions, cut into 2-inch lengths
- 4 teaspoons extra-virgin olive oil
- 2 garlic cloves, thinly sliced
- ½ teaspoon dried rosemary
- ½ teaspoon salt
- 4 (6-ounce) skinless halibut fillets
- ¼ teaspoon freshly ground black pepper
- 3 tablespoons fresh lemon juice

Heat the oven to 450°F.

On a large rimmed baking sheet, toss the asparagus, mushrooms, and scallions with the oil, garlic, rosemary, and ¼ teaspoon of the salt. Roast for 5 minutes.

Push the vegetables to the 2 long edges of the baking sheet and place the halibut in the center. Season the fish with the remaining ¼ teaspoon salt and sprinkle with the pepper and lemon juice. Roast for about 10 minutes longer, until the fish just flakes when tested with a fork and the vegetables are tender. Serve hot.

NUTRITION AT A GLANCE
Per serving: 287 calories, 9 g fat, 1 g saturated fat, 39 g protein, 14 g carbohydrate, 3 g fiber, 389 mg sodium

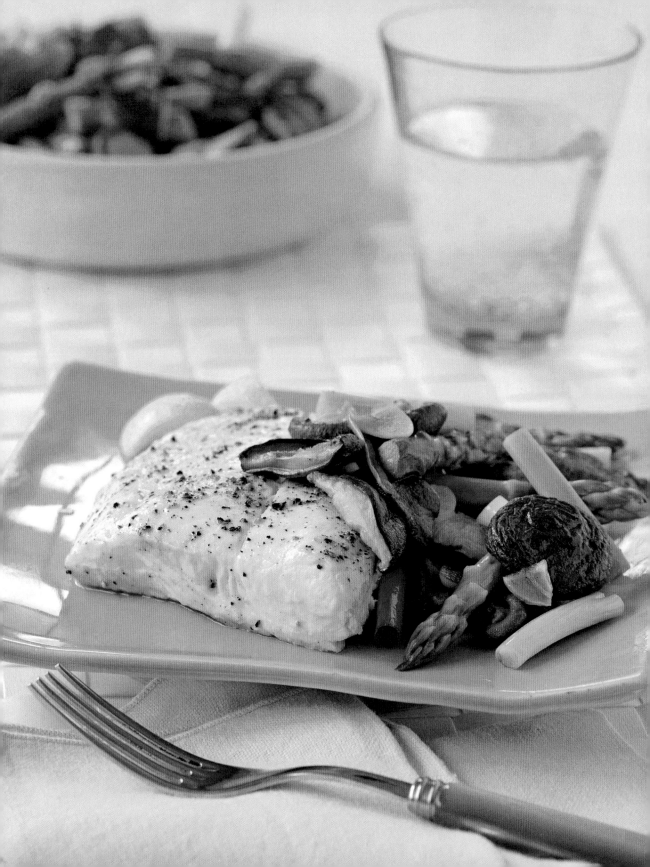

Shrimp Fra Diavolo

MAKES 4 servings   HANDS-ON TIME: 15 minutes   TOTAL TIME: 20 minutes

Classic spicy Shrimp Fra Diavolo (the name means "devilish friar") is usually
served over pasta, but this Phase 1 version is just as delicious without—or serve
over white beans, if you like. See the Variation below for a Phase 2 pasta version.

4 teaspoons extra-virgin olive oil

2 garlic cloves, peeled and halved

1 teaspoon red pepper flakes

1½ pounds peeled and deveined large
   shrimp

¼ teaspoon salt

2 teaspoons anchovy paste, or
   2 anchovies, finely chopped

1 bunch broccoli rabe (12 ounces),
   thinly sliced

2 tablespoons tomato paste

In a large skillet, heat the oil over medium-low heat. Add the garlic and ½ teaspoon
of the red pepper flakes. Cook until the garlic is golden, about 3 minutes.

Increase the heat to medium, add the shrimp, and sprinkle with the salt.
Cook, tossing frequently, until the shrimp turn pink and are just opaque in the
center, about 3 minutes. With a slotted spoon, transfer the shrimp to a bowl and
keep warm.

Add the anchovy paste to the skillet and stir to distribute. Add the
broccoli rabe and remaining ½ teaspoon red pepper flakes. Stir to coat. Add
the tomato paste and 1 cup water to the skillet. Cook, stirring occasionally,
until the broccoli rabe is tender and the sauce thickens, about 5 minutes.

Return the shrimp to the skillet just to reheat. Add salt to taste, if desired.

Divide the shrimp and sauce evenly among 4 plates and serve hot.

NUTRITION AT A GLANCE

Per serving: 259 calories, 9 g fat, 1 g saturated fat, 38 g protein, 6 g carbohydrate, 3 g fiber,
514 mg sodium

Variation: For Phase 2, enjoy the shrimp with pasta: Cook 3 ounces of
whole-wheat angel hair pasta and drain well. Add the shrimp and broccoli
rabe mixture to the pasta and toss to combine.

Per serving (with ½ cup pasta): 339 calories, 9 g fat, 1 g saturated fat, 41 g protein,
22 g carbohydrate, 5 g fiber, 518 mg sodium

Oven "Fried" Fish Sticks

MAKES 4 servings   HANDS-ON TIME: 5 minutes   TOTAL TIME: 15 minutes

15 MINUTE RECIPE

Forget about frozen fish sticks, which are often high in saturated fat! The South Beach Diet version is far healthier and just as tasty. Make sure the oven is nice and hot to ensure a crispy coating that's better than fried.

1   pound skinless mild-flavored white fish fillets, such as sole or perch

2   tablespoons fat-free or 1% milk

1   large egg

⅓   cup whole-wheat cracker crumbs (about 1 ounce)

¼   cup finely grated Parmesan cheese

¼   teaspoon garlic powder

¼   teaspoon paprika

Heat the oven to 400°F. Lightly coat a baking sheet with cooking spray.

Cut the fillets into lengthwise strips, about 1 inch wide.

In a medium bowl, whisk together the milk and egg. In a shallow bowl or pie plate, combine the cracker crumbs, Parmesan, garlic powder, and paprika. Add the fish strips to the egg mixture, turning to coat. Transfer the strips to the bowl with the crumb mixture, again turning to coat.

Arrange the fish on the baking sheet. Bake for 10 minutes, or until the fish just flakes when tested with a fork. Serve hot.

NUTRITION AT A GLANCE

Per serving: 177 calories, 5 g fat, 2 g saturated fat, 26 g protein, 6 g carbohydrate, 1 g fiber, 236 mg sodium

TIP: Be sure to select whole-wheat crackers that don't contain any sugar or trans fats and that provide at least 3 grams of fiber per ounce.

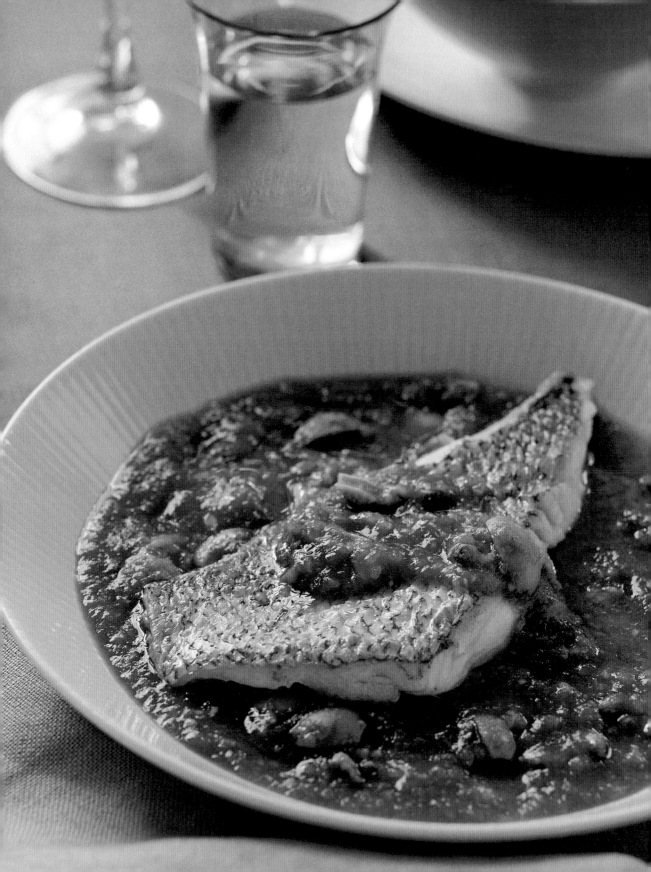

Red Snapper Veracruz

MAKES 4 servings   HANDS-ON TIME: 10 minutes   TOTAL TIME: 20 minutes

Although traditionally made with snapper, this dish also lends itself to other fish, such as tilapia, catfish, and grouper. Keeping the skin on the snapper gives the dish a more colorful presentation.

- 1¼ cups canned diced tomatoes with juice
- 1 medium onion, cut into chunks
- 2 garlic cloves, peeled
- 1 jalapeño pepper, halved and seeded
- ½ teaspoon dried oregano
- ¼ teaspoon dried rosemary
- ½ teaspoon salt
- 4 teaspoons extra-virgin olive oil
- 4 (6-ounce) red snapper fillets, with skin
- ¼ cup pitted green olives, coarsely chopped
- 2 teaspoons nonpareil capers, drained and rinsed

In a blender, combine the tomatoes and their juice, onion, garlic, jalapeño, oregano, rosemary, and ¼ teaspoon of the salt. Purée until smooth.

In a large nonstick skillet, heat the oil over medium heat. Make a few 2-inch cuts in the skin side of the fillets, just through the skin (to prevent the fillets from curling). Season the snapper with the remaining ¼ teaspoon salt. Add the fish to the skillet, skin-side down, and cook until the skin is crisp, about 3 minutes. Transfer the fish to a platter.

In the same skillet, combine the tomato mixture, olives, and capers. Cook until the flavors are combined, 3 minutes. Return the fish to the pan, skin-side up, and cook until the fish just flakes when tested with a fork, 2 minutes longer.

Transfer the fish, skin-side up, to 4 shallow bowls and top evenly with the sauce. Serve hot.

NUTRITION AT A GLANCE
Per serving: 249 calories, 8 g fat, 1 g saturated fat, 36 g protein, 6 g carbohydrate, 1 g fiber, 677 mg sodium

Grouper with Salsa Verde

MAKES 4 servings   HANDS-ON TIME: 10 minutes   TOTAL TIME: 20 minutes

If you can't find grouper for this vibrant recipe, try red snapper, ocean perch, or tilapia. Cilantro stems actually have more flavor than the leaves, so be sure to include some in the salsa, which is just as delicious served with chicken or pork.

8 ounces fresh or canned tomatillos

½ small onion, cut into chunks

1 garlic clove, peeled

½ fresh jalapeño pepper, seeded

4 teaspoons extra-virgin olive oil

⅓ cup cilantro (whole leaves and tender stems)

1 tablespoon fresh lime juice

½ teaspoon salt

4 (6-ounce) skinless grouper fillets

Heat the broiler.

Wash and husk the tomatillos, if using fresh. If using canned, drain well.

In a medium bowl, toss the tomatillos with the onion, garlic, jalapeño, and 2 teaspoons of the oil. Place the mixture on a broiler pan and broil 4 inches from the heat for 3 to 4 minutes, until the tomatillos are softened and lightly charred.

Leaving the broiler on, transfer the tomatillo mixture to a blender or food processor. Add the cilantro, lime juice, and ¼ teaspoon of the salt. Purée until smooth.

Brush the grouper with the remaining 2 teaspoons oil and season with the remaining ¼ teaspoon salt. Transfer to the same broiler pan and broil for 5 minutes, or until the fish is just cooked through and flakes when tested with a fork.

Transfer the fish to 4 plates and top each fillet evenly with the salsa verde. Serve hot.

NUTRITION AT A GLANCE

Per serving: 223 calories, 7 g fat, 1 g saturated fat, 34 g protein, 5 g carbohydrate, 1 g fiber, 383 mg sodium

Baked Tilapia with Toasted Almonds

MAKES 4 servings   HANDS-ON TIME: 10 minutes   TOTAL TIME: 20 minutes

This classic preparation keeps the fish moist while providing a delicious sauce topping. Be sure to keep an eye on the almonds; they can burn quickly if left unattended.

¼ cup sliced almonds	2 teaspoons fresh lemon juice
3 tablespoons mayonnaise	½ teaspoon dried marjoram
1 tablespoon Dijon mustard	½ teaspoon salt
1 teaspoon grated lemon zest	4 (6-ounce) skinless tilapia fillets

Heat the oven to 450°F. In a small ungreased skillet, toast the almonds over medium heat until lightly browned, about 5 minutes.

Meanwhile, in a small bowl, stir together the mayonnaise, mustard, lemon zest, lemon juice, marjoram, and salt. Spread the mixture evenly on the fish. Place the fish on a rimmed baking sheet and scatter the almonds over the tops.

Bake for about 10 minutes, until the topping is golden brown, the almonds are crisp, and the fish flakes easily when tested with a fork. Serve hot.

NUTRITION AT A GLANCE
Per serving: 276 calories, 14 g fat, 2.5 g saturated fat, 35 g protein, 2 g carbohydrate, 1 g fiber, 526 mg sodium

Coconut Shrimp Curry

MAKES 4 servings   HANDS-ON TIME: 20 minutes   TOTAL TIME: 25 minutes

If you have some time and decide to peel and devein the shrimp yourself, you'll need 1½ pounds. Be sure to choose unsweetened lite coconut milk, not the thick sweetened kind used to make piña coladas!

1	cup quick-cooking barley or brown rice	4	teaspoons reduced-sodium soy sauce
1	can (14 ounces) unsweetened lite coconut milk	1¼	pounds peeled and deveined large shrimp
1	tablespoon Thai red curry paste	2	tablespoons fresh lime juice
1	large red bell pepper, slivered	2	tablespoons slivered fresh basil
1	small onion, thinly sliced		Lime wedges, for serving

In a medium saucepan, cook the barley according to package directions. Drain any liquid left in the pan. Cover and keep warm.

Meanwhile, in a medium saucepan, combine 1 cup of the coconut milk and the curry paste. Bring to a simmer over medium heat. Add the bell pepper and onion and cook, stirring often, for 5 minutes to soften the vegetables.

Stir in the soy sauce and remaining coconut milk. Bring to a simmer and cook for 1 minute to blend flavors.

Add the shrimp and cook, stirring often, until the shrimp turn pink and are just opaque in the center, about 5 minutes. Remove from the heat and stir in the lime juice.

Divide the barley among 4 plates, top with the curry, and sprinkle with the basil. Serve with lime wedges for squeezing.

NUTRITION AT A GLANCE
Per serving: 386 calories, 10 g fat, 6 g saturated fat, 36 g protein, 39 g carbohydrate, 5 g fiber, 573 mg sodium

Variation: For Phase 1, serve the shrimp over 1 cup uncooked zucchini (shred it on a box grater) rather than barley.
Per serving (with zucchini instead of barley): 286 calories, 10 g fat, 1 g saturated fat, 39 g protein, 30 g carbohydrate, 6 g fiber, 606 mg sodium

TIP: Look for Thai red curry paste in the Asian section of your supermarket and keep it refrigerated after opening. Different brands vary in spiciness and some can be red hot, so test a little before adding.

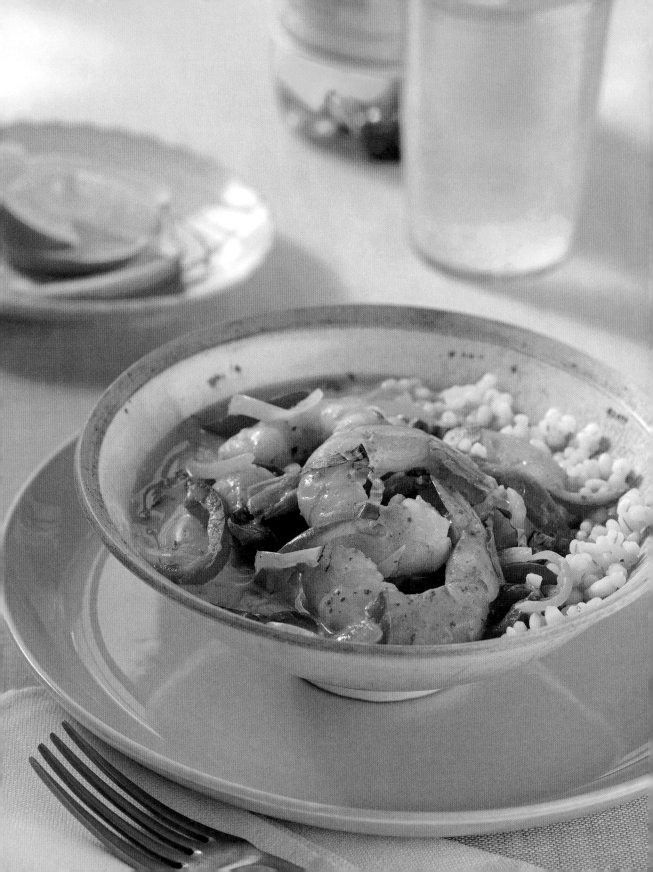

Salmon with White Balsamic Glaze

MAKES 4 servings   HANDS-ON TIME: 5 minutes   TOTAL TIME: 25 minutes

If you've never cooked with white balsamic vinegar, which is now widely available in most grocery stores, you'll enjoy it in this recipe. It is a little less sweet than the darker balsamic and is the perfect addition to a light glaze for salmon.

4 (6-ounce) salmon fillets, with skin	⅓ cup finely chopped red onion
¾ teaspoon salt	½ cup white balsamic vinegar
½ teaspoon dried rosemary, crumbled	2 tablespoons chopped fresh parsley

Heat a large skillet over medium heat. Season the salmon with the salt and rosemary. Place the salmon in the skillet, skin-side down, and cook until the skin is crisp and some of the fat has been released, about 5 minutes.

Turn the salmon skin-side up and cook until the fish just flakes when tested with a fork, about 5 minutes longer. With a slotted spatula, transfer the salmon to a platter, cover, and keep warm.

Add the onion to the pan and cook, stirring frequently, until softened, about 5 minutes.

Stir in the vinegar, increase the heat to high, and cook until slightly reduced, about 3 minutes. Stir in the parsley.

Spoon the sauce over the salmon, divide among 4 plates, and serve warm.

NUTRITION AT A GLANCE
Per serving: 329 calories, 18 g fat, 4 g saturated fat, 34 g protein, 5 g carbohydrate, 0 g fiber, 548 mg sodium

Italian Tuna Burgers

MAKES 4 burgers   HANDS-ON TIME: 15 minutes   TOTAL TIME: 25 minutes

Roasted tomatoes are a great topping for tuna burgers. If you don't have a toaster oven, you can roast the tomatoes on a foil-lined pan under the broiler, 4 to 6 inches from the heat. Use regular whole-wheat bread crumbs and add a little Italian seasoning if whole-wheat Italian bread crumbs are unavailable.

2   plum tomatoes, halved lengthwise

Salt and freshly ground black pepper

1   cup no-salt-added canned chickpeas or cannellini beans, drained and rinsed

2   cans (6 ounces each) water-packed chunk light tuna, very well drained

¼   cup Italian-seasoned whole-wheat bread crumbs (1 ounce)

2   teaspoons grated lemon zest

1   teaspoon fresh lemon juice

2   large egg whites

4   teaspoons extra-virgin olive oil

¼   cup shredded part-skim mozzarella cheese (1 ounce)

4   large slices (1.75 ounces each) whole-wheat peasant bread

4   teaspoons mayonnaise

1   cup baby arugula

Line a toaster-oven tray with foil. Scrape the seeds from the tomato halves. Sprinkle the tomatoes lightly with salt and pepper. Place on the toaster–oven tray and roast at 350° or 400°F (use the higher temperature if the toaster oven is large) just to soften while you make the tuna burgers. Meanwhile, in a large bowl, mash the chickpeas with a potato masher or fork. Add the tuna, bread crumbs, lemon zest, lemon juice, and ¼ teaspoon pepper. Blend well with a fork. Add the egg whites and blend again. Form into 4 patties.

In a large nonstick skillet, heat the oil over medium heat. Add the patties and cook for 5 minutes. Using a spatula, very carefully turn the burgers over and cook on the other side until browned, about 4 minutes longer. Sprinkle each burger with 1 tablespoon mozzarella, cover the pan, and cook for 1 minute longer to melt the cheese.

While the burgers are cooking, toast the bread slices.

Cut the toasted bread slices in half. Spread each of 4 halves with 1 teaspoon mayonnaise. Top each with ¼ cup arugula, a burger, a tomato half, and the remaining bread.

NUTRITION AT A GLANCE
Per burger: 413 calories, 13 g fat, 2 g saturated fat, 31 g protein, 45 g carbohydrate, 8 g fiber, 711 mg sodium

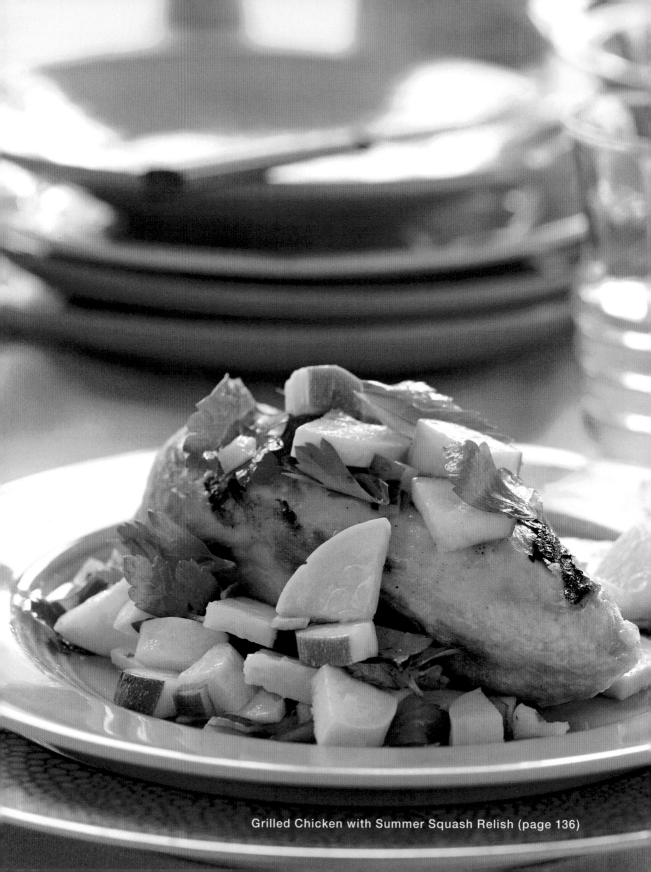

Grilled Chicken with Summer Squash Relish (page 136)

POULTRY

Recipes for chicken are always the most requested by South Beach dieters, and turkey is a close second. It's no wonder, since both types of poultry lend themselves to quick cooking by a variety of methods, from grilling to sautéing to stir-frying. You can now also enjoy skinless, boneless duck breast on all phases of the diet, since the farm-raised breeds, such as Pekin and Magret, are even leaner than chicken when the skin is removed.

What you won't find here is a whole roast chicken. It just takes too long to prepare for a superquick cookbook. Instead there are recipes for burgers made from lean ground chicken and turkey; for chicken and turkey breast cutlets; for stuffed chicken breasts; for mini turkey meatloaves, and more. And even the accompanying sauces and salsas can be made in less than half an hour.

Grilled Chicken with Summer Squash Relish

MAKES 4 servings   HANDS-ON TIME: 10 minutes   TOTAL TIME: 20 minutes

Seasoning the chicken under the skin gives it extra flavor and helps keep it moist (but be sure to discard the skin before serving). If grilling outdoors isn't an option, you can broil the chicken 4 inches from the heat for the same amount of time.

1 teaspoon ground coriander

1 teaspoon ground cumin

¾ teaspoon salt

½ teaspoon ground ginger

¼ teaspoon freshly ground black pepper

4 (10-ounce) bone-in, skin-on chicken breast halves

1 medium yellow squash, quartered lengthwise and thinly sliced

1 medium zucchini, quartered lengthwise and thinly sliced

½ small red onion, finely chopped (⅓ cup)

1 cup whole fresh parsley leaves

2 tablespoons fresh lemon juice

1 tablespoon extra-virgin olive oil

Heat a grill to medium. Lightly oil the grill grates.

Meanwhile, in a small bowl, combine the coriander, cumin, ½ teaspoon of the salt, the ginger, and pepper. With your fingers, carefully lift the chicken skin without removing it. Rub the spice mixture under the skin and pat the skin back down.

Grill the chicken, turning it over halfway through cooking, for about 15 minutes, or until cooked through but still juicy. Let cool slightly.

While the chicken is cooking, in a medium bowl, toss together the yellow squash, zucchini, onion, parsley, lemon juice, oil, and remaining ¼ teaspoon salt until well combined.

When the chicken is cool enough to handle, remove and discard the skin. Serve the chicken warm or at room temperature with the squash relish spooned evenly on top.

NUTRITION AT A GLANCE

Per serving: 204 calories, 7 g fat, 1 g saturated fat, 29 g protein, 7 g carbohydrate, 2 g fiber, 516 mg sodium

Turkey Romesco

MAKES 4 servings   HANDS-ON TIME: 10 minutes   TOTAL TIME: 30 minutes

Romesco is a flavorful red pepper, almond, and garlic sauce that's particularly popular in Spain as a topping for grilled spring onions. Here, its smoky sweetness pairs well with paprika-coated turkey.

1½ pounds boneless, skinless turkey breast for London broil (see Tip)

1½ teaspoons paprika

¾ teaspoon salt

4 teaspoons extra-virgin olive oil

¼ cup natural whole almonds

1 garlic clove, peeled

½ cup roasted red peppers (from a jar), drained and rinsed

1 tablespoon tomato paste

2 teaspoons red wine vinegar

Heat the oven to 450°F. Tuck under the thin ends of the turkey so it's all the same thickness. Season on both sides with the paprika and ½ teaspoon of the salt. Coat with 2 teaspoons of the oil. Place the turkey in a small roasting pan and roast for 10 minutes.

Add ½ cup water to the pan and roast for 10 minutes longer, or until the turkey is cooked through and an instant-read thermometer registers 155°F. Tent the breast with foil (the temperature will rise as the turkey sits and the juices recede into the meat).

While the turkey is resting, in a small skillet, heat the remaining 2 teaspoons oil over low heat. Add the almonds and garlic. Cook until the garlic is golden and the almonds are fragrant, about 5 minutes. Transfer to a blender or food processor and add the peppers, tomato paste, vinegar, remaining ¼ teaspoon salt, and ¼ cup water. Purée until well combined.

Thinly slice the turkey and serve with the romesco sauce.

NUTRITION AT A GLANCE
Per serving: 299 calories, 11 g fat, 1 g saturated fat, 44 g protein, 4 g carbohydrate, 2 g fiber, 630 mg sodium

TIP: In the market, look for turkey breast labeled "for London broil," which means it is cut to a rectangular shape that will cook quickly. If you can't find one, just use a regular 1½-pound piece.

Cook Once, Eat Twice

Double the romesco sauce, then heat the extra and toss it with chickpeas, whole-wheat pasta, and handfuls of arugula for Phase 2.

Southwestern Skillet Turkey

MAKES 4 (1½-cup) servings   HANDS-ON TIME: 25 minutes   TOTAL TIME: 25 minutes

A stir-fry is a great way to work more lean turkey into your diet. Here, strips of turkey cutlet cook quickly and maintain their juiciness. Jícama adds a pleasant crunch. For more on jícama, see page 80.

4 teaspoons extra-virgin olive oil

1 pound turkey breast cutlets, cut crosswise into ½-inch-wide strips

1 teaspoon ground cumin

¼ teaspoon cayenne pepper

1 (½-pound) jícama, peeled and cut into thin matchsticks

1 medium sweet onion, cut into very thin half-rings

Salt

2 cups cherry tomatoes, halved

⅓ cup chopped fresh cilantro

In a large nonstick skillet, heat the oil over medium–high heat. Add the turkey and sprinkle with the cumin and cayenne. Cook, stirring, until the spices are fragrant, 30 seconds. Stir in the jícama, onion, and salt to taste. Cover and cook for 3 minutes to slightly wilt the onion. Stir in the cherry tomatoes, cover, and cook for 2 minutes longer.

Uncover, stir, and cook for another 2 minutes to concentrate the liquid in the bottom of the pan. Stir in the cilantro and serve hot.

NUTRITION AT A GLANCE

Per serving: 213 calories, 6 g fat, 1 g saturated fat, 30 g protein, 11 g carbohydrate, 2 g fiber, 111 mg sodium

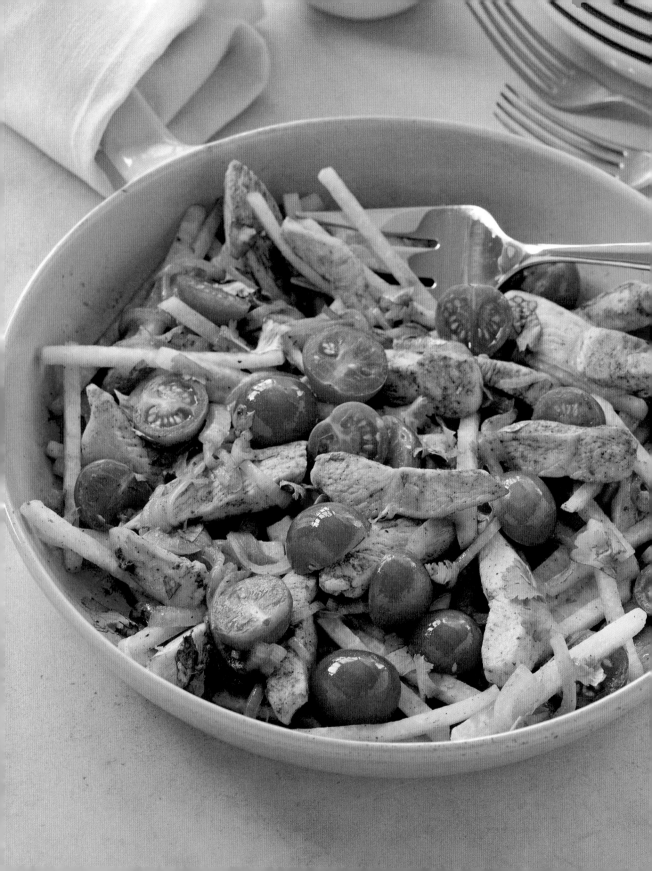

Chicken with Cremini Cream Sauce

MAKES 4 servings   HANDS-ON TIME: 10 minutes   TOTAL TIME: 25 minutes

Cremini mushrooms, also known as brown or Italian mushrooms, are a more flavorful variety of the button mushroom. They come in a range of sizes; try to find small ones for this elegant dish.

4   (6-ounce) boneless, skinless chicken breasts

¾   teaspoon salt

¼   teaspoon freshly ground black pepper

3   teaspoons extra-virgin olive oil

8   ounces small cremini mushrooms, quartered

3   scallions, thinly sliced

½   cup lower-sodium chicken broth

2   tablespoons reduced-fat cream cheese

¼   teaspoon dried rosemary

Season the chicken with ½ teaspoon of the salt and the pepper.

In a large nonstick skillet, heat 2 teaspoons of the oil over medium heat. Add the chicken and cook until golden brown, about 3 minutes per side. Transfer to a plate and keep warm.

Add the mushrooms, scallions, and remaining 1 teaspoon oil to the skillet. Cook over medium heat, tossing frequently, until the mushrooms have wilted, about 3 minutes.

Add the broth, cream cheese, rosemary, and remaining ¼ teaspoon salt. Stir until the cream cheese melts, about 1 minute.

Return the chicken to the pan and bring to a simmer. Cover and cook until the chicken is cooked through and still juicy, about 5 minutes.

Divide the chicken and sauce evenly among 4 plates and serve hot.

NUTRITION AT A GLANCE
Per serving: 256 calories, 7 g fat, 2 g saturated fat, 42 g protein, 4 g carbohydrate, 1 g fiber, 594 mg sodium

Mini Turkey Meatloaves

MAKES 4 meatloaves   **HANDS-ON TIME:** 10 minutes   **TOTAL TIME:** 30 minutes

You make your own fresh bread crumbs from multigrain bread for these individual quick-cooking meatloaves, which are delicious right out of the oven, at room temperature, or chilled for a grab-and-go lunch the next day. Use a mini food processor for speeding up the bread crumb job.

1¼ pounds extra-lean ground turkey breast

2 slices multigrain bread (1 ounce each), chopped to very fine crumbs

¼ cup grated Parmesan cheese

¼ cup sun-dried tomatoes (in oil), drained and minced, plus 1 teaspoon oil from the jar

4 scallions, minced

1 large egg

2 tablespoons tomato paste

1 teaspoon cider vinegar

Heat the oven to 425°F. Line a rimmed baking sheet with foil or parchment.

In a large bowl, combine the turkey, bread crumbs, Parmesan, sun-dried tomatoes, scallions, egg, and 1 tablespoon of the tomato paste. Blend well and form into 4 small loaves 4 inches long and 2 inches wide.

In a small bowl, blend the sun-dried tomato oil with the remaining 1 tablespoon tomato paste, the vinegar, and 2 teaspoons water.

Place the meatloaves on the baking sheet and brush the tops with the tomato paste mixture. Bake for 18 minutes, or until cooked through but still juicy. Serve warm.

NUTRITION AT A GLANCE
Per meatloaf: 256 calories, 7 g fat, 2 g saturated fat, 41 g protein, 11 g carbohydrate, 3 g fiber, 255 mg sodium

Cook Once, Eat Twice

Make extra and crumble the cooked meatloaves into your favorite tomato sauce to toss with whole-wheat pasta.

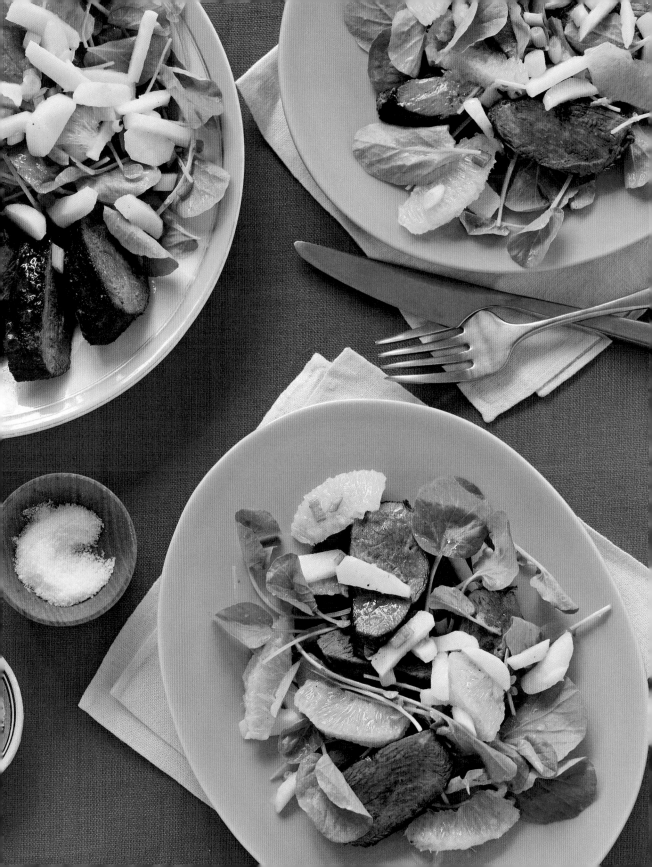

Pan-Grilled Duck Breasts with Orange Salsa

MAKES 4 servings   HANDS-ON TIME: 10 minutes   TOTAL TIME: 15 minutes

Duck breast without the skin is actually leaner than chicken, so it's a great food to enjoy on any phase of the South Beach Diet. Cook these tender breasts just as you would steak and not beyond medium-rare for the best flavor and texture.

- 1 teaspoon mild to medium chili powder
- 1 teaspoon ground cinnamon
- ½ teaspoon ground ginger
- ¾ teaspoon salt
- 4 (5- to 6-ounce) skinless, boneless duck breast halves, all skin removed (see Tip)

- 4 teaspoons extra-virgin olive oil
- 2 navel oranges
- 2 scallions, thinly sliced
- ¼ cup sliced water chestnuts, cut into thin strips
- ½ teaspoon Dijon mustard
- 2 cups watercress, trimmed

In a small bowl, combine the chili powder, cinnamon, ginger, and ½ teaspoon of the salt. Rub the mixture into both sides of the duck breasts and then rub with 2 teaspoons of the oil.

Heat a grill pan over medium heat. Grill the duck until medium-rare, about 3 minutes per side. Let stand for 5 minutes.

Meanwhile, with a paring knife, remove a small slice from the top and bottom of each orange. Following the curve of the fruit, remove the zest and white pith underneath. Segment the oranges, halving the segments, if large.

Transfer the orange segments to a large bowl. Add the scallions, water chestnuts, mustard, remaining 2 teaspoons oil, and remaining ¼ teaspoon salt. Toss to combine.

Thinly slice the duck breasts crosswise. Place ½ cup watercress on each of 4 plates, top with a sliced duck breast, and spoon salsa evenly over the top.

NUTRITION AT A GLANCE
Per serving: 213 calories, 9 g fat, 2 g saturated fat, 22 g protein, 11 g carbohydrate, 2 g fiber, 538 mg sodium

TIP: Most duck breasts come with the fatty skin on. To remove it, simply run a very sharp paring knife between the skin and the breast, using your fingers to gradually pull the skin off.

Crispy Chicken Fingers

MAKES 4 servings   HANDS-ON TIME: 15 minutes   TOTAL TIME: 20 minutes

Kids will love these tasty chicken strips on their own. For an older crowd, they're great served with Baby Greens and Grilled Asparagus with Shallot Vinaigrette (page 224) or Mango Salsa (page 227). You can season the bread-crumb mixture with any of your favorite herbs or spices.

1¼ pounds boneless, skinless chicken breasts	½ teaspoon salt
2 large eggs	¼ teaspoon freshly ground black pepper
½ cup whole-wheat bread crumbs	2 tablespoons extra-virgin olive oil
½ cup whole-wheat flour	1 lemon, cut into wedges, for serving

Place the chicken breasts between 2 pieces of parchment or waxed paper. Using a meat pounder or small heavy skillet, pound to an even ½-inch thickness. Cut the chicken across the grain into 16 (¾-inch-wide) strips.

In a shallow bowl, whisk the eggs. In a separate shallow bowl, combine the bread crumbs, flour, salt, and pepper. Working 1 piece at a time, dip both sides of the chicken strips into the egg mixture and then into the crumb mixture, patting to help the coating adhere. Place the strips on a wire rack as you work.

In a large (12-inch) nonstick skillet, heat the oil over medium heat until very hot but not smoking. Add the chicken strips and cook until golden brown and crisp on the outside and juicy on the inside, about 4 minutes per side. Serve hot with lemon wedges for squeezing.

NUTRITION AT A GLANCE

Per serving: 383 calories, 12 g fat, 2 g saturated fat, 40 g protein, 26 g carbohydrate, 4 g fiber, 584 mg sodium

TIP: If you can't find dried whole-wheat bread crumbs, make your own: Toast a slice or two of whole-wheat bread and pulse in a food processor until fine crumbs form.

Cook Once, Eat Twice

Make a double batch but cook only half of the coated pieces. Freeze the rest on a baking sheet and then pack in a plastic container or resealable plastic bag to cook at a later date.

Cheesy Chicken Tostadas

MAKES 4 servings **HANDS-ON TIME:** 20 minutes **TOTAL TIME:** 25 minutes

This is a main-course cousin of the appetizer Chicken Tostaditas on page 47. You can use any reduced-fat cheese you like (try jalapeño Jack). If you want a smokier flavor, replace the chili powder with 1 tablespoon of minced chipotle in adobo.

4 (8-inch) whole-wheat tortillas	1 teaspoon chili powder
5 teaspoons extra-virgin olive oil	1 teaspoon ground cumin
Salt	½ teaspoon ground coriander
1 pound thin-sliced chicken breast cutlets, cut into very thin strips	½ cup shredded reduced-fat Cheddar cheese (2 ounces)
⅓ cup minced onion	½ avocado, peeled and sliced
1 can (14.5 ounces) diced tomatoes, well drained in a strainer	Fresh cilantro leaves, for garnish (optional)

Heat the oven to 400°F. Line a rimmed baking sheet with foil.

Place the tortillas on the baking sheet. Using a pastry brush, lightly coat the tortillas on 1 side with 1 teaspoon of the olive oil, then sprinkle lightly with salt. Bake the tortillas for 10 minutes, or until lightly browned and crisp. Remove from the oven and turn the oven to broil. Leave the tortillas on the baking sheet.

While the tortillas are baking, in a large nonstick skillet, heat the remaining 4 teaspoons oil over medium-high heat. Add the chicken and onion and sprinkle lightly with salt. Cook, tossing occasionally, until the chicken is almost cooked through, about 3 minutes.

Add the tomatoes, chili powder, cumin, and coriander. Cook, stirring occasionally, until most of the liquid evaporates, about 6 minutes.

Top the tortillas evenly with the chicken mixture, then sprinkle evenly with the cheese. Broil 6 inches from the heat, watching carefully to prevent the tortillas from burning, just until the cheese melts. Top evenly with the avocado and garnish with cilantro, if using. Serve warm.

NUTRITION AT A GLANCE
Per serving: 342 calories, 13 g fat, 3 g saturated fat, 34 g protein, 26 g carbohydrate, 4 g fiber, 530 mg sodium

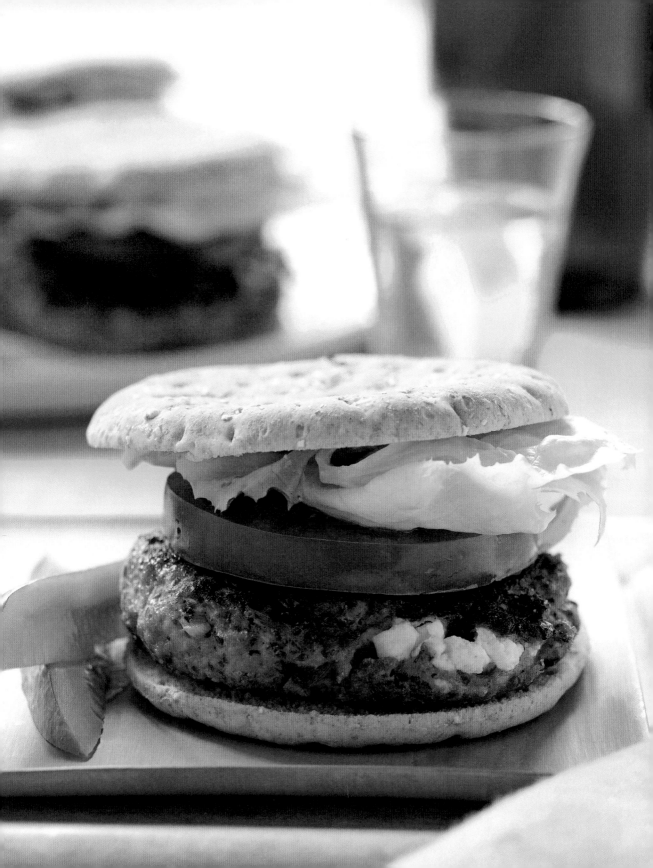

Inside-Out Cheeseburgers

MAKES 4 servings   HANDS-ON TIME: 10 minutes   TOTAL TIME: 20 minutes

These unique cheese-stuffed burgers feature flaxmeal, which is high in cholesterol-lowering soluble fiber and heart-healthy alpha-linolenic acid (ALA). If you can only find whole flaxseed at the market, simply grind it into meal in a spice grinder or small coffee grinder. If you're skipping the bun, just sprinkle a little balsamic on top of the tomato.

1¼ pounds lean ground turkey	4 teaspoons extra-virgin olive oil
½ cup flaxmeal (2 ounces)	4 very thin whole-wheat sandwich rolls (1.5 ounces each), split, or 8 slices multigrain bread (optional)
½ small red bell pepper, finely diced	
2 scallions, thinly sliced	1 tablespoon balsamic vinegar
6 tablespoons reduced-fat soft goat cheese, preferably one flavored with herbs or garlic	4 thick slices tomato
	Bibb lettuce (optional)
¾ teaspoon salt	

In a large bowl, combine the turkey, flaxmeal, bell pepper, scallions, 2 tablespoons of the goat cheese, and ½ teaspoon of the salt. Using your hands, blend well and form into 4 balls. Poke a hole into the center of each ball and stuff each with 1 tablespoon of the remaining goat cheese. Pinch the turkey mixture to seal in the cheese and gently form into 4 patties. Make them as flat as you can (to speed the cooking), taking care not to squeeze the cheese out.

In a large nonstick skillet, heat the oil over medium-high heat. Sprinkle the pan with the remaining ¼ teaspoon salt. Reduce the heat to medium, add the patties, and cook until browned on 1 side, about 3 minutes. Turn the patties over and cook for 2 minutes longer. Add ¼ cup water to the pan, reduce the heat to a high simmer, and cover. Cook for 8 to 10 minutes, until the burgers are cooked all the way through.

Meanwhile, lightly toast the sandwich rolls, if using.

To serve, brush 1 side of each of 4 roll halves with the balsamic vinegar. Top with a burger, a tomato slice, lettuce (if using), and the other roll half.

NUTRITION AT A GLANCE

Per serving (with roll): 371 calories, 11 g fat, 1 g saturated fat, 46 g protein, 28 g carbohydrate, 9 g fiber, 832 mg sodium

Per serving (without roll): 278 calories, 10 g fat, 1 g saturated fat, 42 g protein, 8 g carbohydrate, 4 g fiber, 597 mg sodium

Chicken Cutlets Puttanesca

MAKES 4 servings   HANDS-ON TIME: 15 minutes   TOTAL TIME: 20 minutes

Sometimes making your own tomato sauce takes only a few minutes longer than warming a prepared sauce, and it's ultimately more delicious. This succulent meal of chicken topped with a traditional olive- and caper-infused tomato sauce will become a family favorite.

4 (5-ounce) thin-sliced chicken breast cutlets

Salt and freshly ground black pepper

4 teaspoons extra-virgin olive oil

5 garlic cloves, minced

1 can (28 ounces) crushed tomatoes, with juice

⅓ cup pitted kalamata olives, chopped

2 tablespoons nonpareil capers, drained and rinsed

¼ teaspoon red pepper flakes

¼ cup chopped fresh basil, plus basil leaves for garnish

1 tablespoon fresh lemon juice

Season the chicken cutlets with salt and pepper.

In a large nonstick skillet, heat 2 teaspoons of the oil over medium-high heat. Add the cutlets and cook until lightly browned and cooked through but still juicy, about 3 minutes per side. Transfer to a plate and cover to keep warm.

In the same skillet, heat the remaining 2 teaspoons oil over medium heat. Add the garlic and cook, stirring, for 30 seconds. Add the tomatoes and their juice, olives, capers, and pepper flakes. Bring to a simmer and cook until the sauce is slightly thickened, about 5 minutes.

Stir in the chopped basil and lemon juice. Return the chicken to the pan briefly just to reheat. Serve the chicken hot with the puttanesca sauce on top, garnished with basil leaves.

NUTRITION AT A GLANCE

Per serving: 285 calories, 8 g fat, 1 g saturated fat, 37 g protein, 15 g carbohydrate, 4 g fiber, 606 mg sodium

Variation: For Phase 2, serve each portion of chicken and sauce over ½ cup whole-wheat couscous.

Per serving (with couscous): 313 calories, 7 g fat, 1 g saturated fat, 37 g protein, 19 g carbohydrate, 2 g fiber, 99 mg sodium

Peppered Chicken Cutlets

MAKES 4 servings   **HANDS-ON TIME: 20 minutes**   **TOTAL TIME: 20 minutes**

The combination of white and black pepper makes this chicken dish quite spicy. You might want to try it first with half the pepper called for and see if it is to your taste, or not spicy enough. Look for white pepper that comes in individual grinder jars so you can coarsely grind it yourself. If you can't find it, just use a smaller amount of regular ground white pepper.

- 1 tablespoon coarsely ground white pepper
- 1 teaspoon coarsely ground black pepper
- 4 (5-ounce) thin-sliced chicken breast cutlets
- Salt
- 4 teaspoons extra-virgin olive oil
- 1 cup lower-sodium chicken broth
- 2 tablespoons fresh lemon juice
- 2 tablespoons reduced-fat cream cheese (1 ounce), cut into small pieces

In a shallow bowl or pie plate, combine the white and black pepper. Coat both sides of the cutlets lightly with the pepper mixture, pressing it in to be sure it adheres. Season both sides of the cutlets lightly with salt.

In a large nonstick skillet, heat the oil over medium–high heat. Add the chicken and cook until lightly browned and cooked through but still juicy, about 3 minutes per side. Transfer the chicken to a plate and cover to keep warm.

Add the broth and lemon juice to the skillet and bring to a boil over high heat. Boil until reduced by half, 3 to 4 minutes.

Remove the pan from the heat and whisk in the cream cheese until it melts. Transfer the chicken to 4 plates and top each with about 3 tablespoons sauce.

NUTRITION AT A GLANCE
Per serving: 230 calories, 8 g fat, 2 g saturated fat, 35 g protein, 3 g carbohydrate, 1 g fiber, 144 mg sodium

Quick Turkey Tagine

MAKES 4 (1½-cup) servings **HANDS-ON TIME: 15 minutes** **TOTAL TIME: 15 minutes**

Named for the pot this Moroccan-style dish is traditionally cooked in, a tagine is essentially a stew, often containing fruit. Both sun-dried tomatoes and prunes give this quick-cooking version deep flavor.

Scant 1½ cups boiling water

1 cup whole-wheat couscous

2 teaspoons extra-virgin olive oil

2 garlic cloves, slivered

1 teaspoon ground coriander

1 teaspoon ground ginger

¾ teaspoon salt

¼ teaspoon freshly ground black pepper

1½ cups lower-sodium chicken broth

2 cups frozen butternut squash chunks

⅓ cup sun-dried tomato halves (not oil-packed), thinly sliced

¼ cup pitted prunes, coarsely chopped

1½ pounds boneless, skinless turkey breast, cut into 1-inch chunks

⅓ cup cilantro leaves, chopped

Pour the boiling water over the couscous, stir, cover, and let steam for 7 minutes. Uncover and fluff the couscous with a fork.

Meanwhile, in a large saucepan, heat the oil over medium heat. Add the garlic, coriander, ginger, salt, and pepper. Cook for 1 minute. Add the broth and bring to a boil. Add the squash, sun-dried tomatoes, and prunes. Cook for 5 minutes for the flavors to develop.

Add the turkey, reduce the heat to a simmer, and cook until the turkey is cooked through and still juicy, about 4 minutes.

Stir the cilantro into the turkey mixture and serve warm over the couscous.

NUTRITION AT A GLANCE
Per serving: 384 calories, 4 g fat, 1 g saturated fat, 48 g protein, 39 g carbohydrate, 6 g fiber, 644 mg sodium

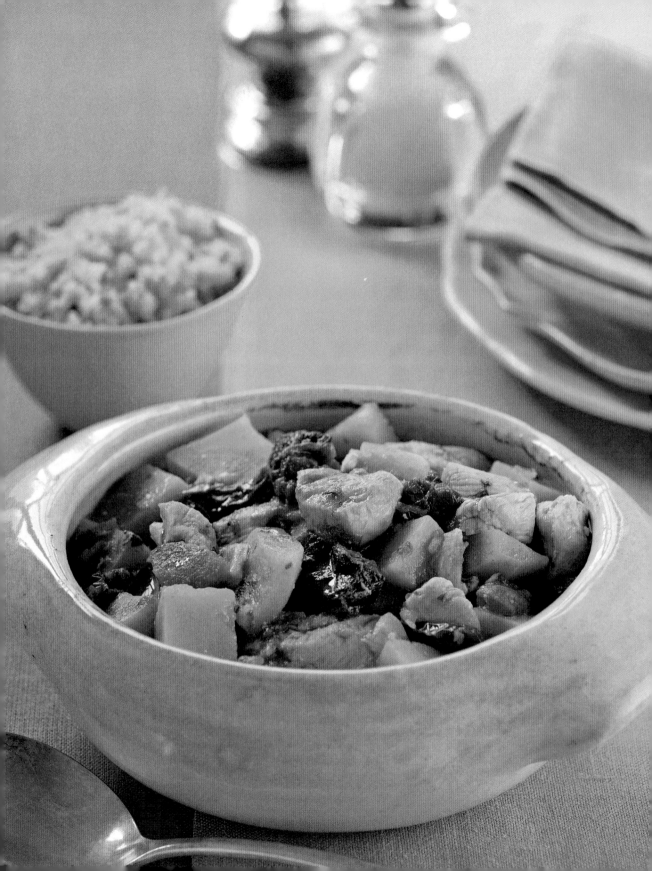

Satay Chicken Burgers

MAKES 4 burgers   HANDS-ON TIME: 15 minutes   TOTAL TIME: 30 minutes

You want the true peanut flavor of a traditional satay sauce to permeate these burgers, so use the peanutty-est natural peanut butter you can find. A brand with a little salt and even a tiny bit of molasses or agave nectar added won't hurt your diet and will add more flavor than one that includes just peanuts. By melting the peanut butter before mixing it with the chilled chicken, you assure that it gets well distributed.

¼ cup natural peanut butter

1¼ pounds ground chicken breast

4 scallions, minced

¼ cup minced fresh cilantro

2 teaspoons grated lemon zest

2 tablespoons fresh lemon juice

1 tablespoon minced pickled jalapeño pepper

¼ teaspoon salt

¼ teaspoon freshly ground black pepper

4 teaspoons extra-virgin olive oil

Bibb lettuce leaves, for serving

Place the peanut butter in a medium metal bowl and set the bowl over a pan of very hot water. Stir just until the peanut butter is just barely liquidy, about 30 seconds. Remove the bowl from the heat.

Add the chicken and mix well to evenly distribute the peanut butter. Sprinkle the scallions, cilantro, lemon zest, lemon juice, jalapeño, salt, and black pepper evenly over chicken and mix well. Form the mixture into 4 patties.

In a large nonstick skillet, heat the oil over medium heat. Add the patties and cook for 5 minutes on one side. Turn the patties over, cover, and cook on the other side for 7 to 8 minutes longer, until opaque throughout. Serve the burgers on lettuce leaves.

NUTRITION AT A GLANCE

Per burger: 277 calories, 13 g fat, 2 g saturated fat, 34 g protein, 6 g carbohydrate, 2 g fiber, 329 mg sodium

Variation: If you're on Phase 2, enjoy the burger on a whole-grain bun.

Per serving (with bun): 389 calories, 16 g fat, 2 g saturated fat, 38 g protein, 25 g carbohydrate, 3 g fiber, 526 mg sodium

Chicken Milanese

MAKES 4 servings   HANDS-ON TIME: 10 minutes   TOTAL TIME: 25 minutes

Our version of traditional Italian Veal Milanese (in which a hot breaded veal chop is topped with a cool salad) features chicken breasts. Use a good-quality Parmesan, such as Reggiano, for the coating. It will make the dish richer tasting.

½ cup old-fashioned rolled oats

¼ cup grated Parmesan cheese (1 ounce)

¼ teaspoon salt

1 large egg white

4 (6-ounce) boneless, skinless chicken breast halves

2 tablespoons extra-virgin olive oil

1 teaspoon trans-fat-free margarine (vegetable oil spread)

1 tablespoon red wine vinegar

2 teaspoons Dijon mustard

Freshly ground black pepper

8 cups mixed field greens (8 ounces)

3 plum tomatoes, each cut into 8 wedges

In a mini food processor, grind the oats to the texture of dried bread crumbs. Add the Parmesan and salt and pulse to combine. Transfer to a shallow bowl or pie plate. In another shallow bowl, beat the egg white with 1 tablespoon water.

Dip the chicken in the egg white and then in the oat mixture, patting to help the coating adhere.

In a large nonstick skillet, heat 1 tablespoon of the oil and the margarine over medium-high heat. Add the chicken and cook for 5 minutes. Reduce the heat to medium, turn the chicken, and cook on the second side until cooked through but still juicy, 10 to 12 minutes.

Meanwhile, in a large bowl, whisk together the remaining 1 tablespoon oil, the vinegar, and mustard. Season with pepper to taste. Add the mixed greens and toss well.

Place a chicken breast on each of 4 plates. Top each with one-fourth of the greens and 6 tomato wedges.

NUTRITION AT A GLANCE
Per serving: 356 calories, 12 g fat, 3 g saturated fat, 46 g protein, 13 g carbohydrate, 4 g fiber, 444 mg sodium

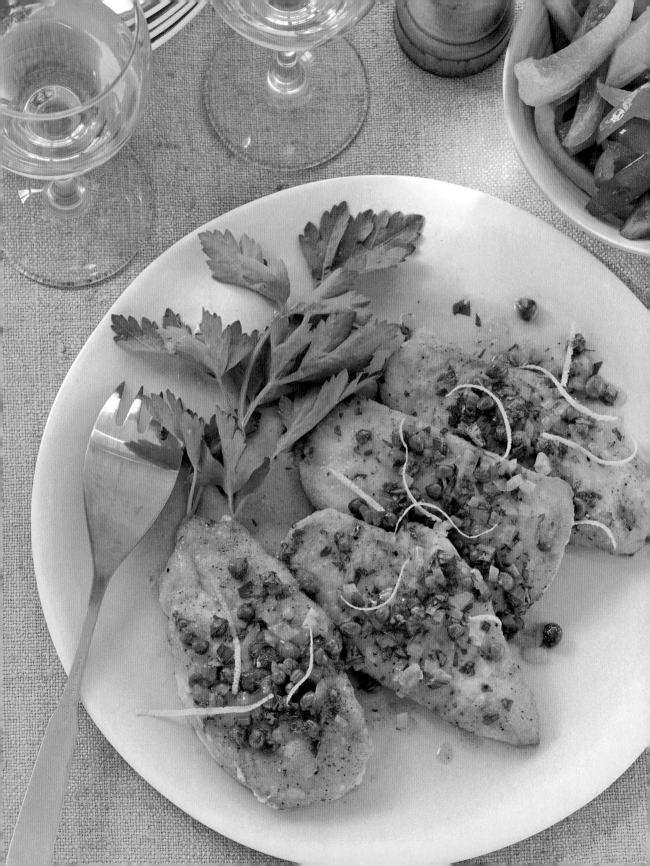

Lemon-Caper Chicken

MAKES 4 servings   HANDS-ON TIME: 15 minutes   TOTAL TIME: 15 minutes

If you want to double this recipe and make it for eight, use two skillets. Or, you can just as easily halve it for a more intimate dinner. Serve the chicken with crispy and colorful red and yellow bell pepper strips or Roasted Green and Wax Beans with Walnuts (page 211).

4 (5-ounce) thin-sliced chicken breast cutlets

Salt and freshly ground black pepper

4 teaspoons whole-wheat flour

1 tablespoon extra-virgin olive oil

1 medium shallot, minced

2 tablespoons capers, drained and rinsed

½ cup lower-sodium chicken broth

¼ cup fresh lemon juice

2 tablespoons minced fresh parsley

Lemon twists, for garnish (optional)

Season the chicken with salt and pepper, then lightly coat with the flour, using about 1 teaspoon for each breast.

In a large nonstick skillet, heat the oil over medium-high heat. Add the chicken and cook until lightly browned and cooked through but still juicy, about 3 minutes per side. Transfer the chicken to a serving platter, cover, and keep warm.

Add the shallot and capers to the skillet and cook over low heat, stirring, for 30 seconds. Add the broth and lemon juice and cook, stirring, until incorporated and thickened, about 1 minute. Stir in the parsley and immediately pour the sauce over the chicken. Serve warm, garnished with lemon twists if you like.

NUTRITION AT A GLANCE
Per serving: 174 calories, 5 g fat, 2 g saturated fat, 27 g protein, 4 g carbohydrate, 1 g fiber, 212 mg sodium

Goat Cheese and Arugula–Stuffed Chicken Breasts

MAKES 4 servings   HANDS-ON TIME: 20 minutes   TOTAL TIME: 25 minutes

For the creamiest filling, choose soft goat cheese over the firmer varieties. If you can't find arugula, substitute baby spinach. Serve the chicken with Warm Mushroom Salad with Toasted Pecans (page 209) and Chocolate Meringue Kisses (page 264) for dessert.

- 2 ounces soft reduced-fat goat cheese, cut into pieces
- 1 garlic clove, minced
- 4 (6-ounce) boneless, skinless chicken breast halves
- 1 bunch arugula (3 ounces), trimmed and coarsely chopped
- Salt and freshly ground black pepper
- 1 tablespoon extra-virgin olive oil
- ¾ cup lower-sodium chicken broth

In a small bowl, stir together the cheese and garlic.

Using a sharp knife, cut a horizontal slit through the thickest portion of each chicken breast to form a deep pocket. Stuff each pocket with an equal amount of the cheese mixture and the arugula. Press the edges of the pocket together to seal. Season the chicken with salt and pepper.

In a large nonstick skillet, heat the oil over medium-high heat. Add the chicken and cook for 4 minutes per side, or until lightly browned. Reduce the heat to medium. Add the broth, cover, and simmer for about 6 minutes, until the chicken is just cooked through and still juicy. With a slotted spatula transfer to 4 serving plates. Serve hot.

NUTRITION AT A GLANCE
Per serving: 255 calories, 8 g fat, 2 g saturated fat, 43 g protein, 2 g carbohydrate, 0.5 g fiber, 181 mg sodium

Chicken with Wine-Braised Mushrooms

MAKES 4 servings   HANDS-ON TIME: 25 minutes   TOTAL TIME: 30 minutes

This traditional bistro offering combines mushrooms, shallots, and white wine in a quick, savory topping for chicken breasts (the alcohol evaporates, which makes this fine for Phase 1).

4 (5-ounce) boneless, skinless chicken breast halves	½ cup dry white wine or chicken broth
Salt and freshly ground black pepper	1 tablespoon fresh lemon juice
4 teaspoons extra-virgin olive oil	½ teaspoon dried tarragon
12 ounces white mushrooms, sliced	Parsley leaves, for garnish
1 small shallot, minced	

Season the chicken all over with salt and pepper.

In a large nonstick skillet, heat 2 teaspoons of the oil over medium–high heat. Add the chicken and cook until browned on one side, about 3 minutes. Turn and cook on the other side for 4 minutes longer, or until the chicken is cooked through and still juicy. Transfer to a plate.

Heat the remaining 2 teaspoons oil in the skillet over medium heat. Add the mushrooms and shallot and cook, stirring occasionally, until the mushrooms start to soften, about 5 minutes.

Add the wine, lemon juice, and tarragon and cook, stirring, for 3 minutes. Return the chicken to the pan, cover, and cook for 2 minutes longer.

Top the chicken with the mushrooms and garnish with parsley leaves.

NUTRITION AT A GLANCE
Per serving: 243 calories, 7 g fat, 1 g saturated fat, 34 g protein, 4 g carbohydrate, 0 g fiber, 99 mg sodium

Variation: If you're on Phase 2, serve the chicken and mushrooms atop ½ cup whole-wheat couscous.
Per serving (with couscous): 313 calories, 7 g fat, 1 g saturated fat, 37 g protein, 19 g carbohydrate, 2 g fiber, 99 mg sodium

TIP: Shallots impart a savory flavor to the wine sauce. Make sure you select bulbs that are firm, dry, and sprout-free. Store them for up to a month in a cool, dry, well-ventilated place or in a covered container in the fridge.

Chicken Tri-Colore

MAKES 4 (1¾-cup) servings   HANDS-ON TIME: 25 minutes   TOTAL TIME: 25 minutes

Vitamin-rich bell peppers provide the three bright colors in this festive dish. Add an orange pepper too, if you like.

1½ pounds boneless, skinless chicken breasts, cut into ½-inch chunks

¾ teaspoon salt

½ teaspoon dried oregano

¼ teaspoon freshly ground black pepper

2 tablespoons extra-virgin olive oil

3 garlic cloves, peeled

1 medium green bell pepper, cut into thin strips

1 medium red bell pepper, cut into thin strips

1 medium yellow bell pepper, cut into thin strips

2 bunches arugula, each bunch trimmed and cut in half crosswise

2 tablespoons balsamic vinegar

In a large bowl, toss the chicken with ½ teaspoon of the salt, the oregano, and black pepper.

In a large nonstick skillet, heat 1 tablespoon of the oil over low heat. Add the garlic and cook until fragrant, about 3 minutes. With a slotted spoon, remove the garlic and discard.

Increase the heat to medium. Add half of the chicken. Cook, turning occasionally, until golden brown and cooked through, about 4 minutes. With a slotted spoon, transfer to a plate. Repeat with the remaining oil and chicken.

Add all the bell peppers and the remaining ¼ teaspoon salt to the skillet. Cook over medium heat, stirring frequently, until the peppers are crisp-tender, about 4 minutes.

Add the arugula and cook, tossing, until wilted, about 1 minute. Return the chicken to the pan, sprinkle with the vinegar, and toss to combine. Serve hot.

NUTRITION AT A GLANCE
Per serving: 288 calories, 9 g fat, 2 g saturated fat, 41 g protein, 8 g carbohydrate, 2 g fiber, 555 mg sodium

Cook Once, Eat Twice
Double the recipe and serve as a salad, chilled or at room temperature.

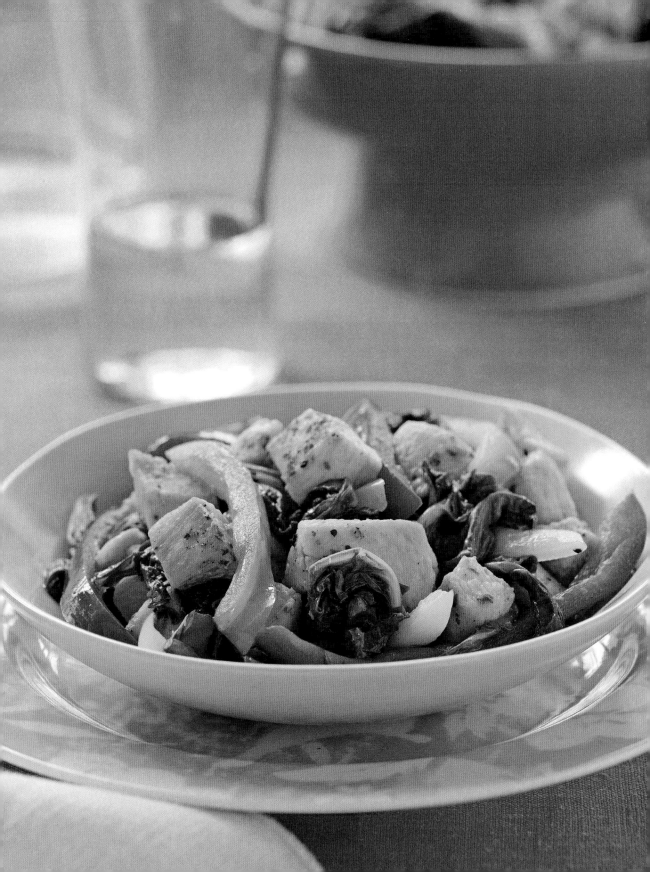

Chicken Dijonnaise with Tomato-Scallion Relish

MAKES 4 servings HANDS-ON TIME: 10 minutes TOTAL TIME: 20 minutes

If you can't find thin-sliced chicken breast cutlets, buy regular chicken breasts and use a meat pounder or small heavy skillet to flatten them to a uniform thickness so they'll cook more quickly. Be sure to zest the lemon before you squeeze the juice. You can also grill the chicken on an outdoor grill.

¼ cup low-fat plain yogurt

2 tablespoons Dijon mustard

1 tablespoon fresh lemon juice

1 teaspoon dried tarragon

4 (5-ounce) thin-sliced chicken breast cutlets

8 ounces cherry tomatoes, coarsely chopped

3 scallions, thinly sliced

2 teaspoons grated lemon zest

Salt and freshly ground black pepper

Heat the broiler. Line a broiler pan with foil.

In a shallow bowl, combine the yogurt, mustard, lemon juice, and tarragon. Add the chicken cutlets one at a time and turn to coat. Transfer to the broiler pan and let stand while you prepare the relish.

In a medium bowl, combine the tomatoes, scallions, lemon zest, and salt and pepper to taste.

Broil chicken 6 inches from the heat for 5 minutes per side, or until cooked through but still juicy.

Serve the chicken topped with the tomato-scallion relish.

NUTRITION AT A GLANCE
Per serving: 189 calories, 2 g fat, 1 g saturated fat, 34 g protein, 6 g carbohydrate, 1 g fiber, 288 mg sodium

TIP: A Microplane zester, which looks like a carpenter's rasp with a plastic handle, makes quick work of zesting lemons and limes.

Chicken with Spicy Roasted Tomato-Leek Sauce

MAKES 4 servings   HANDS-ON TIME: 10 minutes   TOTAL TIME: 30 minutes

This versatile dish is good either hot or chilled. Trim off the darkest portions of the leeks' green tops as well as the rootlets at the base. And be sure to rinse the leeks well after halving, since soil and grit can collect in between the layers.

1½ pounds cherry tomatoes

3 leeks, halved lengthwise, rinsed well, and cut crosswise into 1-inch pieces

4 teaspoons extra-virgin olive oil

2 garlic cloves, smashed and peeled

2 tablespoons fresh tarragon leaves or 1 teaspoon dried

¾ teaspoon red pepper flakes

¾ teaspoon salt

4 (6-ounce) boneless, skinless chicken breast halves

Heat the oven to 425°F. On a rimmed baking sheet, toss the tomatoes and leeks with 3 teaspoons of the oil, the garlic, tarragon, pepper flakes, and ½ teaspoon of the salt. Roast for 10 minutes, tossing once.

Meanwhile, season the chicken with the remaining ¼ teaspoon salt and remaining 1 teaspoon oil.

Nestle the chicken on the pan among the leeks and tomatoes. Return to the oven and roast for 10 minutes longer, or until the chicken is just cooked through and still juicy.

Divide the chicken and vegetables among 4 plates and serve hot.

NUTRITION AT A GLANCE
Per serving: 305 calories, 7 g fat, 1 g saturated fat, 42 g protein, 17 g carbohydrate, 3 g fiber, 569 mg sodium

Cook Once, Eat Twice
Double the recipe. The next day, chop the remaining leek and tomato mixture, add some olives and capers, and serve this "dressing" over the cold sliced chicken breast.

Roast Chicken with Chili-Lime Sauce

MAKES 4 servings   HANDS-ON TIME: 5 minutes   TOTAL TIME: 30 minutes

Keeping the skin on the chicken while it roasts preserves moistness at the high cooking temperature and allows the herb mixture to penetrate the meat (be sure to remove the skin before serving). Olive oil rather than flour or another starch helps to thicken the uncooked sauce, making it an ideal Phase 1 recipe.

2 teaspoons herbes de Provence	1 tablespoon fresh lime juice
½ teaspoon salt	¾ teaspoon chili powder
4 (10-ounce) bone-in, skin-on chicken breast halves	1 tablespoon extra-virgin olive oil
⅓ cup tomato juice	

Heat the oven to 425°F.

In a small bowl, combine the herbes de Provence and ¼ teaspoon of the salt. With your fingers, carefully lift the chicken skin without removing it. Rub the herbes de Provence mixture under the skin and over the chicken.

Place the chicken on a rimmed baking sheet. Roast for 25 minutes, or until cooked through but still juicy. Let cool briefly. When cool enough to handle, remove and discard the skin.

Meanwhile, in another small bowl, whisk together the tomato juice, lime juice, chili powder, and remaining ¼ teaspoon salt. Whisk in the oil.

Divide the chicken among 4 plates. Drizzle each serving with 2 tablespoons sauce and serve warm.

NUTRITION AT A GLANCE
Per serving: 197 calories, 5 g fat, 1 g saturated fat, 34 g protein, 1 g carbohydrate, 0 g fiber, 603 mg sodium

TIP: Herbes de Provence is a blend of dried herbs that typically contains thyme, basil, rosemary, marjoram, fennel seed, anise seed, lavender, and savory. Look for it in small packets at your supermarket, or make your own blend, combining equal parts of these herbs.

Five-Spice Grilled Chicken with Asian Dipping Sauce

MAKES 4 servings   HANDS-ON TIME: 10 minutes   TOTAL TIME: 20 minutes

This versatile chicken can be served hot, at room temperature, or chilled and would make a nice base for an Asian-inspired salad. Five-spice powder, a combination of cinnamon, ground cloves, fennel seed, star anise, and Szechuan peppercorns, flavors the chicken.

2¼ teaspoons five-spice powder

¼ teaspoon salt

4 (6-ounce) boneless, skinless chicken breast halves

4 teaspoons extra-virgin olive oil

6 tablespoons rice vinegar

3 tablespoons reduced-sodium soy sauce

2 (2-inch) pieces fresh ginger, grated (no need to peel)

2 garlic cloves, minced

In a large shallow bowl, stir together the five-spice powder and salt. Add the chicken breasts and rub the mixture into them. Add the oil and toss to coat.

Heat a grill pan over medium-high heat. Place the chicken on the pan and grill until cooked through and still juicy, about 4 minutes per side. Transfer to a plate, cover with foil, and let stand for 5 minutes.

While the chicken is cooking, in a small bowl, whisk together the vinegar and soy sauce. With your hands, squeeze the grated ginger over the bowl, extracting as much juice as possible into the vinegar mixture. Add the garlic to the sauce and stir to combine.

Slice the chicken on a diagonal. Transfer to 4 plates and serve with small bowls of the sauce (about 2 tablespoons each) for dipping.

NUTRITION AT A GLANCE
Per serving: 262 calories, 7 g fat, 1 g saturated fat, 40 g protein, 8 g carbohydrate, 0 g fiber, 690 mg sodium

Cook Once, Eat Twice

Double the recipe and refrigerate the extra chicken and sauce separately. The next day, slice the chicken and toss it with shredded napa cabbage, peanuts, a little tofu, and the sauce.

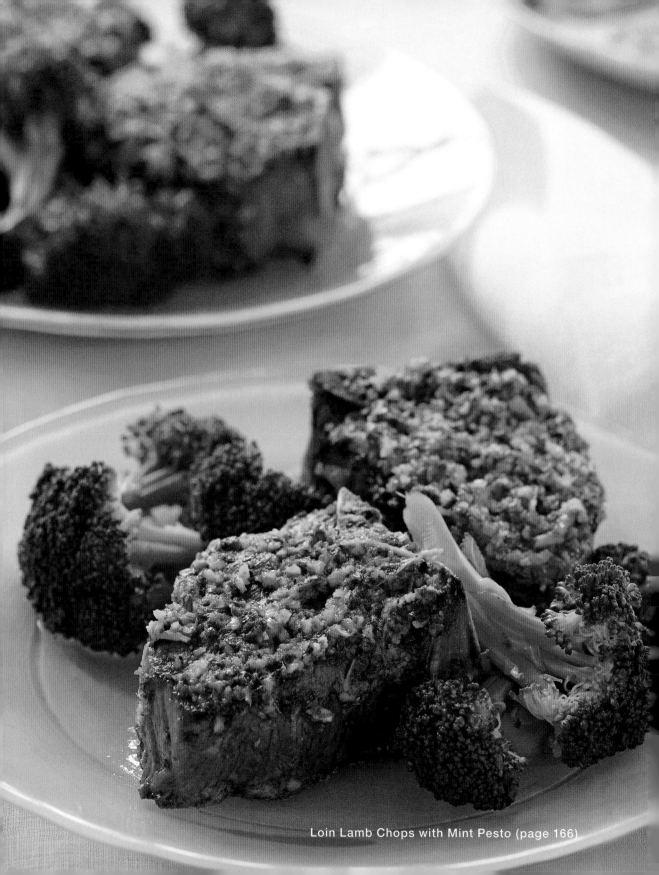

Loin Lamb Chops with Mint Pesto (page 166)

MEATS

Today beef, lamb, and pork are leaner than ever—and a mainstay of the South Beach Diet if you enjoy them. Here we transform the quickest-cooking cuts—pork loin, loin lamb chops, flank steak, sirloin—into rich-tasting dishes with sauces like chimichurri, cashew, and watercress cream. If your budget allows it, look for grass-fed beef and lamb, which are lower in overall fat and saturated fat and have the added advantage of providing more heart-healthy omega-3 fatty acids than meat from conventionally raised animals.

For fast preparation, make sure you have a sharp chef's knife and meat pounder (see page 12). You'll want the chef's knife to butterfly the pork loin for the soft pork tacos recipe and the pounder to flatten the pork for the 15-minute piccata, the spicy pork skewers, and the roasted pork with sweet and sour cucumbers.

Loin Lamb Chops with Mint Pesto

MAKES 4 servings (2 chops each)   HANDS-ON TIME: 10 minutes   TOTAL TIME: 15 minutes

The mint pesto that accompanies these lamb chops is so much healthier than the sugary mint jelly that's often served. Because loin lamb chops are lean and tiny, you'll want two for each serving. The chops are broiled to save time, but you could pan-sear them in batches if you prefer. They're delicious served with steamed broccoli, Brussels sprouts, or another dark green vegetable.

MINT PESTO

- ⅔ cup packed fresh mint leaves
- ¼ cup packed fresh parsley leaves
- 2 tablespoons pine nuts or chopped walnuts
- 1 garlic clove, smashed and peeled
- ½ teaspoon grated lemon zest
- 1 tablespoon fresh lemon juice
- 1 tablespoon extra-virgin olive oil

LAMB CHOPS

- 8 loin lamb chops (each about 1 inch thick), well trimmed

  Salt and freshly ground black pepper

Heat the broiler.

For the pesto: In a blender or food processor, process the mint, parsley, nuts, garlic, lemon zest, and lemon juice until finely chopped. With the machine running, drizzle in the oil and process until almost smooth.

For the lamb: Place the chops on a broiler pan. Season lightly with salt and pepper. Broil the chops for 3 minutes per side for medium-rare.

Transfer 2 chops to each of 4 plates and top evenly with the pesto.

NUTRITION AT A GLANCE

Per serving: 253 calories, 14 g fat, 4 g saturated fat, 28 g protein, 2 g carbohydrate, 1 g fiber, 92 mg sodium

Spicy Pork Skewers with Cashew Sauce

MAKES 4 (6-skewer) servings   HANDS-ON TIME: 15 minutes   TOTAL TIME: 20 minutes

These pork skewers are a variation on the traditional Southeast Asian satay—grilled meat, poultry, or seafood that is dipped into a spicy peanut sauce. Here, more flavorful cashews are the base for the sauce instead of peanuts.

- 8 teaspoons reduced-sodium soy sauce
- 2 teaspoons hot pepper sauce
- 1 teaspoon extra-virgin olive oil
- 6 (4-ounce) thin-cut boneless pork loin chops, well trimmed

- 2 large garlic cloves, unpeeled
- 3 ounces unsalted toasted cashews (scant ¾ cup)
- 1 tablespoon fresh lime juice
- Lime wedges, for serving

Heat the broiler. Line a broiler pan with foil.

In a large bowl, combine 4 teaspoons of the soy sauce, the hot pepper sauce, and oil.

Cut each piece of pork lengthwise into 4 strips. Place the strips between 2 pieces of parchment or waxed paper. With a meat pounder or small, heavy skillet, pound the strips to about a ¼-inch thickness. Add the pork to the soy sauce mixture and let marinate while you make the cashew sauce.

In a small saucepan of boiling water, cook the garlic for 1 minute and remove. When cool enough to handle, peel and place in a mini food processor with the remaining 4 teaspoons soy sauce, the cashews, lime juice, and ½ cup water. Process to a smooth purée.

Thread the pork strips onto 24 (6- to 8-inch) wooden or metal skewers and place on the broiler pan. Broil 6 inches from the heat, without turning, for 4 minutes, or until the pork is cooked through but still juicy.

Divide the pork skewers among 4 plates and serve with individual bowls of the cashew sauce (about 2½ tablespoons each) and lime wedges for squeezing.

NUTRITION AT A GLANCE
Per serving: 312 calories, 17 g fat, 4 g saturated fat, 30 g protein, 10 g carbohydrate, 1 g fiber, 516 mg sodium

Cook Once, Eat Twice

Double the recipe and turn half into a second-day pork salad: Cut the cooked pork into bite-size pieces and toss with the cashew sauce, along with halved grape or cherry tomatoes, mixed greens, and a little more lime juice.

15 MINUTE RECIPE

Grilled Sirloin Steaks with Shallot-Mustard Sauce

MAKES 4 servings   HANDS-ON TIME: 5 minutes   TOTAL TIME: 10 minutes

The simple sauce for these steaks could also be made with a grainy Dijon mustard, and with red wine vinegar in place of the lemon juice. The sauce is equally delicious on grilled chicken or pork.

4 (4- to 5-ounce) boneless sirloin steaks

½ teaspoon salt

½ teaspoon freshly ground black pepper

4 teaspoons extra-virgin olive oil

1 tablespoon Dijon mustard

2 tablespoons fresh lemon juice

1 large shallot, finely chopped

Heat a grill pan over medium heat or heat the broiler with the rack 4 inches from the heat source. Season the steaks on both sides with the salt and pepper.

Brush the steaks with 1 teaspoon of the oil. Grill the steaks or broil on a broiler pan for 3 to 4 minutes per side for medium-rare.

Meanwhile, in a small bowl whisk the together the remaining 3 teaspoons oil, the mustard, lemon juice, and shallot.

Divide the steaks among 4 plates and drizzle evenly with the sauce.

NUTRITION AT A GLANCE
Per serving: 207 calories, 10 g fat, 3 g saturated fat, 25 g protein, 3 g carbohydrate, 0 g fiber, 446 mg sodium

Cook Once, Eat Twice

Double the recipe and turn the extra into a steak salad (or a sandwich on Phase 2), using the extra shallot-mustard sauce as a dressing or spread. Or, just make a double batch of the sauce for a dressing to be drizzled over cold chicken or pork.

Pork Piccata

MAKES 4 servings   **HANDS-ON TIME:** 15 minutes   **TOTAL TIME:** 15 minutes

15 MINUTE RECIPE

A typical Italian-style piccata is made with veal or chicken. Here, the piquant lemon-wine piccata sauce complements lean pork chops. Whisking a little trans-fat-free margarine into the sauce instead of the usual butter is a healthy way to add richness without saturated fat.

- 4 (4-ounce) boneless center-cut pork loin chops, well trimmed
- 2 tablespoons whole-wheat flour
- ½ teaspoon salt
- ¼ teaspoon freshly ground black pepper
- 1 tablespoon extra-virgin olive oil

- ⅓ cup dry white wine
- 3 tablespoons fresh lemon juice
- 1 teaspoon trans-fat-free margarine (vegetable oil spread)
- 2 tablespoons chopped fresh parsley

Place the pork chops between 2 pieces of parchment or waxed paper. With a meat pounder or small heavy skillet, pound to a ¼-inch thickness.

In a shallow bowl or pie plate, blend the flour, salt, and pepper. Dredge the pork in the seasoned flour, shaking off the excess.

In a large nonstick skillet, heat the oil over medium-high heat. Add the pork and cook quickly until cooked through but still juicy, about 1 minute per side. Transfer to a plate and cover to keep warm.

Add the wine and lemon juice to the skillet. Simmer over medium heat, stirring to get up the browned bits, until the sauce is reduced by half, about 2 minutes. Remove the pan from the heat and whisk in the margarine. Stir in the parsley.

Divide the warm cutlets among 4 plates and spoon 1 tablespoon sauce on top of each.

NUTRITION AT A GLANCE
Per serving: 208 calories, 9 g fat, 2 g saturated fat, 25 g protein, 3 g carbohydrate, 0.4 g fiber, 221 mg sodium

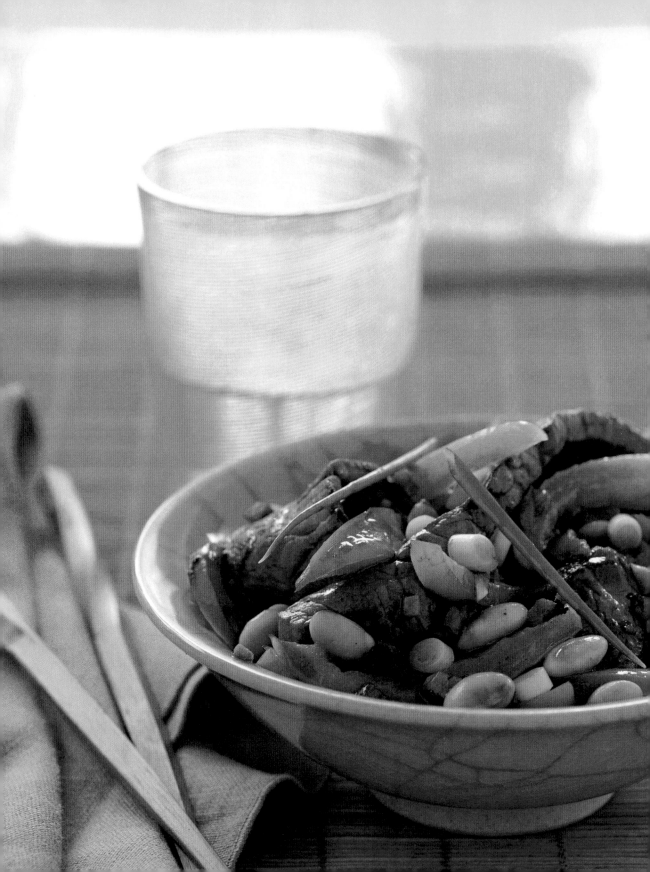

Ginger Beef and Edamame Stir-Fry

MAKES 4 (1½-cup) servings   HANDS-ON TIME: 15 minutes   TOTAL TIME: 15 minutes

A superflavorful stir-fry is a fast and tasty dinner solution on a busy weeknight. Cutting the round steak thinly across the grain makes it more tender. Here we use orange bell pepper, but you can use any color pepper you like.

1½ pounds bottom round steak, well trimmed

2 teaspoons dark sesame oil

3 large garlic cloves, minced

2 tablespoons minced fresh ginger

2 tablespoons reduced-sodium soy sauce

1 teaspoon cornstarch

1 cup frozen shelled edamame

½ cup thinly sliced orange bell pepper

2 scallions, thinly sliced

Slice the beef across the grain into ¼-inch-thick slices.

In a large nonstick skillet or wok, heat the sesame oil over high heat until almost smoking. Add the garlic and ginger and cook, stirring constantly, until fragrant, about 30 seconds. Add the beef and cook, stirring occasionally, until lightly browned, about 5 minutes.

Meanwhile, in a small bowl, combine the soy sauce, cornstarch, and 3 tablespoons water.

Add the edamame, bell pepper, and scallions to the beef mixture. Cook, stirring, until heated through, about 1 minute. Add the soy sauce mixture and cook until the sauce thickens, about 2 minutes. Divide evenly among 4 plates and serve hot.

NUTRITION AT A GLANCE

Per serving: 344 calories, 15 g fat, 4 g saturated fat, 42 g protein, 7 g carbohydrate, 3 g fiber, 400 mg sodium

Lamb Porcupines

MAKES 4 servings (2 meatballs each) HANDS-ON TIME: 10 minutes TOTAL TIME: 25 minutes

These meatballs are called porcupines because the rice protrudes once the lamb is cooked. They're a healthier variation of a classic Betty Crocker meatball recipe made with beef and white rice. For a change of pace, use a soft reduced-fat goat cheese instead of feta.

- ¾ pound lean ground lamb
- 2 ounces crumbled reduced-fat feta cheese
- ½ cup whole fresh cilantro leaves or mint leaves
- ⅓ cup quick-cooking whole-grain brown rice
- 1 large egg
- ½ teaspoon dried marjoram
- ½ teaspoon salt
- ¼ teaspoon freshly ground black pepper
- 1 can (15 ounces) crushed tomatoes
- 4 tablespoons part-skim ricotta cheese

In a medium bowl, combine the lamb, feta, cilantro, rice, egg, marjoram, salt, pepper, and ¼ cup water. Mix well. Shape into 8 golf ball–size meatballs.

In a large skillet, heat the tomatoes over medium heat. Add the meatballs, cover, and cook for about 15 minutes, until the meat is cooked through and the rice is tender.

Spoon 2 meatballs and some sauce onto each of 4 plates and top each serving with 1 tablespoon ricotta.

NUTRITION AT A GLANCE

Per serving: 355 calories, 23 g fat, 11 g saturated fat, 24 g protein, 15 g carbohydrate, 3 g fiber, 711 mg sodium

Greek Sloppy Joes with Feta and Whole-Wheat Orzo

MAKES 4 servings   HANDS-ON TIME: 20 minutes   TOTAL TIME: 30 minutes

In this Greek–inspired variation of the popular sloppy Joe, whole-wheat orzo takes the place of the traditional white bun.

- 5 ounces whole-wheat orzo (about ¾ cup)
- 4 teaspoons extra-virgin olive oil
- 1 large onion, finely chopped
- 3 garlic cloves, minced
- ¾ pound lean ground sirloin
- 1 teaspoon dried oregano
- ½ teaspoon cayenne pepper
- ½ teaspoon ground cinnamon
- 1 can (14.5 ounces) diced tomatoes, with juice
- 3 tablespoons tomato paste
- 4 tablespoons crumbled reduced-fat feta
- 1 scallion, thinly sliced

Bring a medium saucepan of lightly salted water to a boil. Add the orzo and cook according to the package directions. Drain well.

Meanwhile, in a large nonstick skillet, heat the oil over medium heat. Add the onion and garlic and cook, stirring occasionally, until the onion is soft and beginning to brown, about 5 minutes.

Add the beef and break up with a spoon. Sprinkle with the oregano, cayenne, and cinnamon. Cook until the beef is almost all browned but still a little pink, about 3 minutes.

Stir in the diced tomatoes and their juice, tomato paste, and ¼ cup water. Simmer until the sauce is thickened and flavorful, about 10 minutes.

Divide the orzo evenly among 4 bowls and ladle the beef mixture evenly on top. Sprinkle each with 1 tablespoon feta and some scallion.

NUTRITION AT A GLANCE
Per serving: 328 calories, 10 g fat, 3 g saturated fat, 25 g protein, 37 g carbohydrate, 7 g fiber, 438 mg sodium

Variation: **For Phase 1, simply eliminate the orzo.**
Per serving (without orzo): 217 calories, 10 g fat, 3 g saturated fat, 21 g protein, 15 g carbohydrate, 2 g fiber, 438 mg sodium

Soft Pork Tacos

MAKES 4 servings   **HANDS-ON TIME:** 10 minutes   **TOTAL TIME:** 25 minutes

Butterflying the pork tenderloin is quick and easy to do if you have a good sharp knife (see page 12 for more on knives); otherwise ask the butcher to do it. By almost slicing the tenderloin in half and opening it, you make it much thinner and it roasts that much faster. Using bottled salsa and prepared coleslaw mix also saves time here.

1 (¾-pound) pork tenderloin	½ cup nonfat (0%) plain Greek yogurt
1½ teaspoons ground cumin	1 cup store-bought green salsa
¾ teaspoon salt	4 (8-inch) whole-wheat tortillas
¼ teaspoon freshly ground black pepper	1 cup shredded coleslaw mix
1 teaspoon extra-virgin olive oil	

Heat the oven to 450°F. With a chef's knife, cut the pork almost in half lengthwise without cutting through the bottom and open like a book (this is butterflying). Place the pork on a rimmed baking sheet and rub all over with 1¼ teaspoons of the cumin, ½ teaspoon of the salt, and the pepper. Brush all over with the oil.

Roast the pork for 15 minutes, or until cooked through and still juicy.

Transfer the pork to a plate and tent with foil (the internal temperature will rise as it sits). Let sit for 5 minutes before thinly slicing crosswise.

While the pork is sitting, in a small bowl, stir together the yogurt, remaining ¼ teaspoon cumin, and remaining ¼ teaspoon salt.

In a medium bowl, combine the pork and salsa and toss to coat. Divide among the 4 tortillas, placing the meat in the center. Top evenly with the slaw mix and then the yogurt mixture. Fold 2 opposite edges of each tortilla over the filling, then roll up to enclose.

NUTRITION AT A GLANCE
Per taco: 282 calories, 6 g fat, 1 g saturated fat, 25 g protein, 27 g carbohydrate, 3 g fiber, 725 mg sodium

Flank Steak with Chimichurri

MAKES 4 servings   **HANDS-ON TIME: 5 minutes**   **TOTAL TIME: 15 minutes**

Chimichurri is a popular sauce in Argentina, where it is often served with steak. You can make the chimichurri a day ahead and refrigerate it until ready to use. If you have any sauce left over, try it with slices of ripe tomato.

- 1 tablespoon Dijon mustard
- 4 teaspoons plus 1 tablespoon red wine vinegar
- 4 teaspoons extra-virgin olive oil
- ½ teaspoon salt
- ½ teaspoon ground ginger
- ⅛ teaspoon cayenne pepper

- 1 (1-pound) flank steak
- ½ cup whole cilantro leaves and chopped tender stems
- ½ cup whole fresh parsley leaves
- 1 garlic clove, peeled
- 1 teaspoon ground cumin

Heat the broiler.

In a small bowl, stir together the mustard, 4 teaspoons of the vinegar, 2 teaspoons of the oil, ¼ teaspoon of the salt, the ginger, and half the cayenne.

Place the flank steak on a broiler pan and brush the top with the vinegar mixture. Broil 4 inches from the heat, without turning, for about 7 minutes for medium-rare. Remove from under the broiler and leave the steak on the broiler pan. Cover loosely with foil and let stand for 5 minutes.

While steak is broiling, in a blender, combine the cilantro, parsley, garlic, cumin, remaining 1 tablespoon vinegar, remaining 2 teaspoons oil, remaining ¼ teaspoon salt, remaining cayenne, and 2 tablespoons water. Purée until smooth.

Thinly slice the flank steak on an angle against the grain. Divide the steak among 4 plates and top evenly with the chimichurri. Serve warm.

NUTRITION AT A GLANCE

Per serving: 209 calories, 11 g fat, 3 g saturated fat, 25 g protein, 1 g carbohydrate, 1 g fiber, 359 mg sodium

Cook Once, Eat Twice

Double the recipe and use the extra to make a steak salad, adding watercress and red and yellow grape tomatoes. Or, prepare a bigger batch of the chimichurri and use as a salad dressing.

Pork and Pepper Stew

MAKES 4 (2-cup) servings   HANDS-ON TIME: 20 minutes   TOTAL TIME: 30 minutes

This flavorful stew has a double dose of peppers—green bell pepper as well as pickled jalapeño.

4 teaspoons extra-virgin olive oil	½ cup packed chopped fresh cilantro
1¼ pounds boneless center-cut pork loin chops, well trimmed and cut into 1-inch chunks	1 small pickled jalapeño pepper, finely chopped
1 large green bell pepper, cut into ½-inch chunks	½ teaspoon ground coriander
	½ teaspoon salt
6 scallions, thinly sliced	1 package (10 ounces) frozen green peas, thawed
3 garlic cloves, minced	
2 tablespoons whole-wheat flour	1 tablespoon fresh lime juice
3 cups lower-sodium chicken broth	4 tablespoons shredded reduced-fat Monterey Jack cheese (1 ounce)

In a nonstick Dutch oven, heat the oil over medium-high heat. Add the pork and cook, stirring, for 2 minutes, to just color it. Transfer to a plate. Add the bell pepper, scallions, and garlic to the pan. Stir until the pepper begins to soften, about 3 minutes.

Sprinkle the vegetables evenly with the flour and stir to combine. Gradually stir in the broth. Add the cilantro, jalapeño, coriander, and salt. Return the pork to the pan. Bring to a low boil over high heat. Reduce the heat and simmer until the pork is cooked through, about 5 minutes.

Stir the peas and lime juice into the stew. Divide the stew among 4 bowls and sprinkle each serving with 1 tablespoon shredded cheese.

NUTRITION AT A GLANCE
Per serving: 342 calories, 12 g fat, 3 g saturated fat, 40 g protein, 18 g carbohydrate, 5 g fiber, 617 mg sodium

Variation: Turn this into a Phase 1 recipe by substituting ½ cup canned white beans for the peas and omitting the whole-wheat flour.

Per serving (with beans and without peas and flour): 294 calories, 11.5 g fat, 3 g saturated fat, 37 g protein, 11 g carbohydrate, 1 g fiber, 647 mg sodium

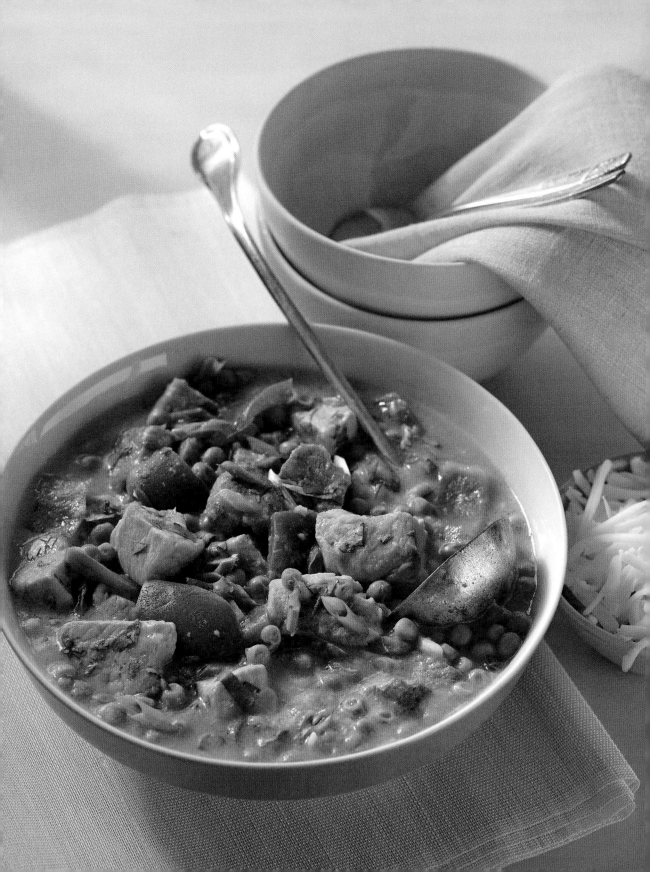

Mushroom-Beef Burgers with Watercress Cream

MAKES 4 burgers HANDS-ON TIME: 15 minutes TOTAL TIME: 25 minutes

These burgers are enhanced by horseradish and watercress, both fiber-rich, heart-healthy cruciferous vegetables.

6 ounces cremini mushrooms, quartered

1¼ pounds lean ground sirloin

2 teaspoons prepared horseradish

Oil, for grill pan

⅓ cup chopped watercress leaves and tender stems

½ cup nonfat (0%) plain Greek yogurt

8 thin slices (1 ounce each) whole-wheat peasant bread (lightly toasted if you like)

In a food processor, finely chop the mushrooms, pulsing on and off, until they are the texture of coarse bread crumbs. Transfer to a medium bowl. Add the beef and horseradish and thoroughly combine. Form into 4 patties, each about 1 inch thick.

Lightly oil a grill pan and heat over medium heat. Place the patties on the pan and cook for 6 minutes per side for medium to medium-rare.

Meanwhile, in a small bowl, stir together the watercress and yogurt.

For each burger, spread 1 slice of bread with 1 tablespoon of the watercress cream. Top with a burger, another 1 tablespoon watercress cream, and the second slice of bread.

NUTRITION AT A GLANCE
Per burger (with bread): 359 calories, 10 g fat, 3 g saturated fat, 38 g protein, 5 g carbohydrate, 5 g fiber, 319 mg sodium

Variation: If you're on Phase 1, simply omit the bread and enjoy the burger on a bed of lettuce (or more watercress).

Per burger (without bread): 201 calories, 8 g fat, 3 g saturated fat, 31 g protein, 3 g carbohydrate, 0 g fiber, 103 mg sodium

Roasted Pork with Sweet and Sour Cucumbers

MAKES 4 servings **HANDS-ON TIME:** 10 minutes **TOTAL TIME:** 30 minutes

Sweet and sour cucumbers are a flavorful alternative to sauerkraut as an accompaniment for pork. Pounding the tenderloin allows it to roast in just 20 minutes.

- 3 tablespoons reduced-sodium soy sauce
- 2 tablespoons tomato paste
- 1 garlic clove, peeled
- 1 (1-pound) pork tenderloin
- 2 small cucumbers

- 2 tablespoons minced red onion
- 2 tablespoons rice vinegar
- 1 teaspoon granular sugar substitute
  Pinch red pepper flakes

Heat the oven to 450°F with an oven rack in the top third. Line a rimmed baking sheet with foil.

In a mini food processor, combine the soy sauce, tomato paste, and garlic. Process to a smooth purée.

Place the pork between 2 pieces of parchment or waxed paper. With a meat pounder or small heavy skillet, pound to a ¾-inch thickness.

Coat 1 side of the pork with about one-third of the purée. Turn and coat liberally with the remaining purée. Place the pork on the baking sheet. Roast for 15 to 20 minutes, until cooked through but still juicy (an instant-read thermometer should register 150°F). Let the pork sit briefly, then thinly slice crosswise.

While the pork is cooking, peel the cucumbers and halve lengthwise. Scrape out the seeds with a spoon and thinly slice the halves crosswise. In a medium bowl, combine the cucumber, onion, vinegar, sugar substitute, and red pepper flakes.

Serve the sliced pork with the cucumbers alongside. If you like, drizzle a little of the liquid from the bowl of cucumbers over the meat.

NUTRITION AT A GLANCE
Per serving: 152 calories, 3 g fat, 1 g saturated fat, 25 g protein, 5 g carbohydrate, 1 g fiber, 500 mg sodium

Cook Once, Eat Twice
Double the recipe and enjoy half as a chilled salad.

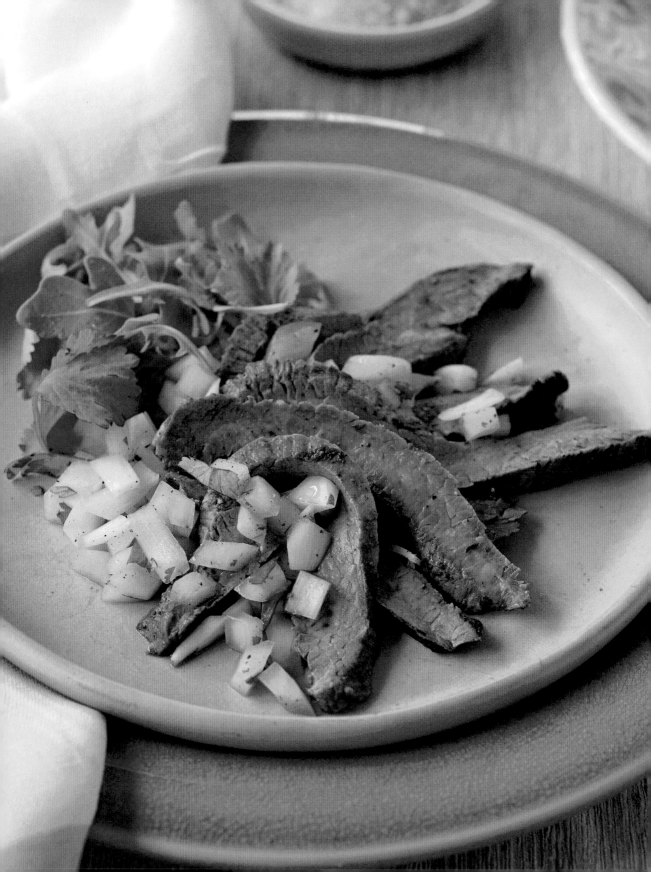

Chili-Rubbed Flank Steak with Sweet Onion Relish

MAKES 4 servings   HANDS-ON TIME: 10 minutes   TOTAL TIME: 30 minutes

Use a Vidalia or another sweet onion for the relish that accompanies this spicy steak. Instead of broiling, you could easily cook the steak on an outdoor grill over medium-high heat for 4 to 5 minutes a side. Keep in mind that flank steak is very lean and will toughen if you overcook it. Enjoy it with a salad of baby greens.

1¼	pounds flank steak		Salt
7	teaspoons fresh lime juice	1	medium sweet onion, minced
2½	teaspoons chili powder	⅓	cup chopped fresh cilantro

Heat the broiler.

Rub both sides of the steak with 2 teaspoons of the lime juice. Sprinkle both sides with 2 teaspoons of the chili powder and rub in. Season lightly with salt. Let sit while you make the onion relish.

In a medium bowl, combine the onion, cilantro, remaining 5 teaspoons lime juice, and remaining ½ teaspoon chili powder (add more chili powder to taste if you like).

Broil the steak 6 inches from the heat for about 6 minutes per side for medium-rare. Transfer to a cutting board and let sit for 5 minutes before thinly slicing at an angle against the grain.

Divide the steak and onion relish evenly among 4 plates and serve warm.

NUTRITION AT A GLANCE
Per serving: 255 calories, 12 g fat, 5 g saturated fat, 31 g protein, 5 g carbohydrate, 1 g fiber, 82 mg sodium

Texas Bowl o' Red

MAKES 4 servings   HANDS-ON TIME: 10 minutes   TOTAL TIME: 25 minutes

This classic Texas dish isn't a chili but rather pieces of meat in a spicy gravy. The "red" in the title doesn't refer to beans or tomatoes, as you might expect, but to the addition of red chiles (in this case in the chili powder and optional chipotle powder). Normally this stew would cook for hours because it's typically made with fatty beef. Made with lean sirloin, it's ready in less than 30 minutes.

2	tablespoons mild chili powder	4	teaspoons extra-virgin olive oil
1	tablespoon chickpea flour or whole-wheat flour	1½	pounds sirloin, well trimmed and cut into 1-inch chunks
1	teaspoon dried oregano	4	garlic cloves, minced
½	teaspoon chipotle chile powder (optional)		

In a small bowl, combine the chili powder, chickpea flour, oregano, and chipotle powder (if using).

In a large nonstick skillet, heat the oil over medium–high heat until very hot but not smoking. Add the beef and garlic and cook, stirring, until the beef is browned on all sides, about 1 minute.

Sprinkle the chili powder mixture over the beef, stirring to coat well. Add ⅔ cup water to the skillet and bring to a boil over high heat. Reduce the heat and simmer, stirring occasionally, for 15 minutes to concentrate the flavors.

Ladle the stew evenly into 4 bowls and serve warm.

NUTRITION AT A GLANCE
Per serving: 282 calories, 13 g fat, 4 g saturated fat, 38 g protein, 2 g carbohydrate, 0 g fiber, 98 mg sodium

Variation: To make this for Phase 1, simply omit the flour.

Per serving (without flour): 276 calories, 13 g fat, 4 g saturated fat, 37 g protein, 1 g carbohydrate, 0 g fiber, 98 mg sodium

TIP: Serve the stew with a crispy coleslaw to cut the spiciness and whole grain bread, if you like, to mop up the sauce.

Pork Tenderloin "Steaks" with Prunes

MAKES 4 servings   HANDS-ON TIME: 5 minutes   TOTAL TIME: 20 minutes

Prunes are a high-fiber addition to the red wine sauce in this delicious pork dish. To make the cooking superquick, the pork tenderloin is cut into medallions, then the medallions are cut open and folded out into thin "steaks."

1 (1-pound) pork tenderloin, cut crosswise into 4 pieces

½ teaspoon salt

½ teaspoon freshly ground black pepper

2 teaspoons extra-virgin olive oil

½ cup dry red wine

¾ cup lower-sodium chicken broth

⅓ cup diced pitted prunes

½ teaspoon rubbed sage

Cut each piece of pork almost in half horizontally, without cutting all the way through. Open up each to form a steak. Season the pork steaks with ¼ teaspoon of the salt and ¼ teaspoon of the pepper.

In a large nonstick skillet, heat the oil over medium–high heat. Add the pork and cook until richly browned, 3 to 4 minutes per side. Transfer to a plate.

Add the wine to the skillet, bring to boil, and boil for 1 minute. Add the broth, prunes, sage, and remaining ¼ teaspoon salt and ¼ teaspoon pepper. Stir in the pork and any juices that have accumulated on the plate. Simmer until the pork is cooked through but still juicy, 3 to 4 minutes.

Transfer a pork steak to each of 4 serving plates. With a potato masher or the back of a spoon, lightly mash some of the prunes to thicken the sauce. Top each steak with 3 tablespoons of the sauce.

NUTRITION AT A GLANCE
Per serving: 224 calories, 5 g fat, 1 g saturated fat, 25 g protein, 14 g carbohydrate, 2 g fiber, 366 mg sodium

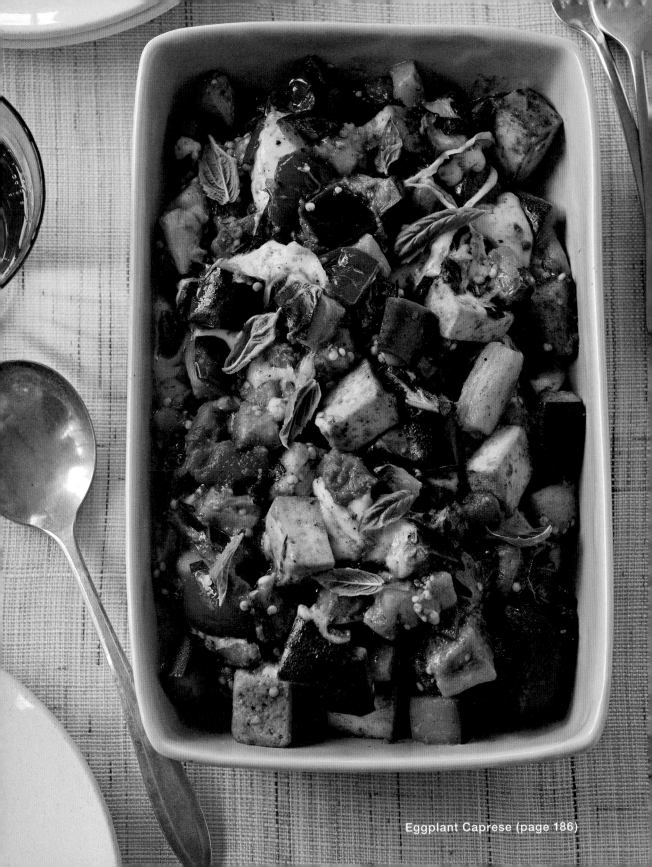

Eggplant Caprese (page 186)

MEATLESS MAINS

You've heard of meatless Mondays, but on the South Beach Diet we advocate serving meatless meals even more often than that. Not only do vegetarian (and vegan) dishes ensure that you're including plenty of high-quality plant protein in your diet, they also suit a tight food budget.

To get your meatless meals on the table in record time, stock your pantry with a variety of whole-wheat pastas and quick-cooking, high-fiber grains, including barley, brown rice, and quinoa, as well as chickpeas, lentils, and all kinds of canned beans. Soy-based meat alternatives, such as tofu, edamame, tempeh, and texturized vegetable protein (TVP) are also essential items for vegetarian meal plans, as are eggs, nuts, and reduced-fat cheeses. Combined with the freshest vegetables, these nutritious foods will assure you always enjoy a satisfying and healthy meal.

Eggplant Caprese

MAKES 4 (1¾-cup) servings   HANDS-ON TIME: 15 minutes   TOTAL TIME: 25 minutes

This spin on the popular Italian salad is a quick-cooking entrée of mozzarella, tomatoes, and basil, along with baked tofu for extra protein. Look for baked tofu where you find tempeh in supermarkets or health-food stores. Rinse off the extra seasonings on the outside, since the tofu is flavored all the way through. If you can't find baked tofu, substitute extra-firm plain tofu.

- 2 teaspoons extra-virgin olive oil
- 1 medium-large eggplant (about 1¼ pounds), cut into 1-inch cubes
- Salt and freshly ground black pepper
- 4 plum tomatoes, cut into ½-inch chunks
- ½ cup shredded fresh basil leaves, plus optional small sprigs for garnish
- 4 ounces baked tofu, preferably with Italian seasonings, cut into ½-inch cubes
- 3 ounces part-skim mozzarella, cut into ½-inch cubes

In a large nonstick skillet, heat the oil over medium-high heat. Add the eggplant and season with salt and pepper to taste. Add ⅓ cup water, cover tightly, and steam for 5 minutes. Stir, add more water if the pan is dry, re-cover, and cook for 4 to 5 minutes, until the eggplant is soft.

Add the tomatoes and shredded basil, stirring to combine. Cover and cook for 2 minutes to heat the tomatoes through and break them down a bit.

Remove the pan from the heat and stir in the tofu and mozzarella. Serve warm, garnished with basil sprigs, if desired.

NUTRITION AT A GLANCE

Per serving: 178 calories, 10 g fat, 3 g saturated fat, 12 g protein, 13 g carbohydrate, 7 g fiber, 245 mg sodium

---

TIP: The fastest way to shred basil is to pile up 8 or 10 leaves, then roll the stack like a cigar. Cut across the roll to shred, or chiffonade, the basil.

Cook Once, Eat Twice

Double the recipe and serve the dish at room temperature the next day. Or, toss with cold whole-wheat pasta or hot couscous and some diced cooked chicken breast for Phase 2.

Individual Pizzas with Gruyère, Caramelized Onions, and Apples

MAKES 4 pizzas   HANDS-ON TIME: 10 minutes   TOTAL TIME: 30 minutes

The combination of apples, cheese, nuts, and rosemary gives an autumnal flavor to these easy pizzas. Gruyère is a nutty cheese that melts easily. You could use reduced-fat Swiss instead.

- 4 teaspoons extra-virgin olive oil
- 2 medium onions, halved and thinly sliced
- 2 medium red apples, halved, cored, and thinly sliced
- 2 cans (15 ounces each) white beans, drained and rinsed
- 2 tablespoons fresh lemon juice
- ½ teaspoon salt
- ¼ teaspoon dried rosemary, crumbled
- 4 (8-inch) whole-wheat tortillas
- 2 cups shredded reduced-fat Gruyère cheese (8 ounces)
- ¼ cup chopped pecans

Heat the oven to 450°F.

In a large skillet, heat 2 teaspoons of the oil over medium heat. Add the onions and toss to coat. Add ¾ cup water, bring to a boil, and cook for 5 minutes longer.

Add the apple slices and cook until the apples are crisp-tender, the onions are golden, and the liquid has evaporated, 7 to 10 minutes.

Meanwhile, in a medium bowl, using a potato masher, mash the beans with the remaining 2 teaspoons oil, the lemon juice, salt, rosemary, and 3 tablespoons water.

Place the tortillas on 2 large baking sheets. Spread the beans evenly over the tortillas. Top evenly with the onion-apple mixture, cheese, and pecans. Bake for about 5 minutes, until the pizzas are piping hot and the cheese has melted. Serve hot.

NUTRITION AT A GLANCE
Per pizza: 648 calories, 24 g fat, 7 g saturated fat, 36 g protein, 78 g carbohydrate, 14 g fiber, 844 mg sodium

15
MINUTE
RECIPE

Cauliflower and Shells in Cheddar Sauce

MAKES 4 (1¼-cup) servings   HANDS-ON TIME: 10 minutes   TOTAL TIME: 15 minutes

Here's a satisfying pasta dish that's not all about the pasta. Pinto beans provide nutritious fiber. For a boost of beta-carotene, look for orange cauliflower at your market. Chickpea flour (see page 67) is used to thicken the sauce; it is lighter and more flavorful than wheat flour.

4 ounces small or medium whole-wheat pasta shells (about 1 cup)

2 cups small cauliflower florets (8 ounces)

1 can (15.5 ounces) pinto beans, drained and rinsed

1 cup 1% or fat-free milk

3 tablespoons chickpea flour

2 teaspoons Dijon mustard

1 cup shredded reduced-fat sharp Cheddar cheese (4 ounces)

Salt and freshly ground black pepper

Chopped fresh chives, for garnish (optional)

Bring a large saucepan of lightly salted water to a boil. Add the pasta and cook according to package directions. Add the cauliflower for last 5 minutes of cooking time. Drain the pasta and cauliflower well and transfer to a serving bowl. Stir in the beans.

As soon as you add the pasta to the boiling water, start the Cheddar sauce: In a small saucepan, stir ¼ cup of the milk into the chickpea flour. Stir in the remaining ¾ cup milk and the mustard. Bring to a simmer over medium-low heat, stirring often. Add the cheese in handfuls, stirring to melt each batch. Season to taste with salt and pepper.

Pour the cheese sauce over the pasta mixture and toss to coat. Garnish with fresh chives if you like.

NUTRITION AT A GLANCE
Per serving: 304 calories, 8 g fat, 4 g saturated fat, 4 g protein, 42 g carbohydrate, 8 g fiber, 490 mg sodium

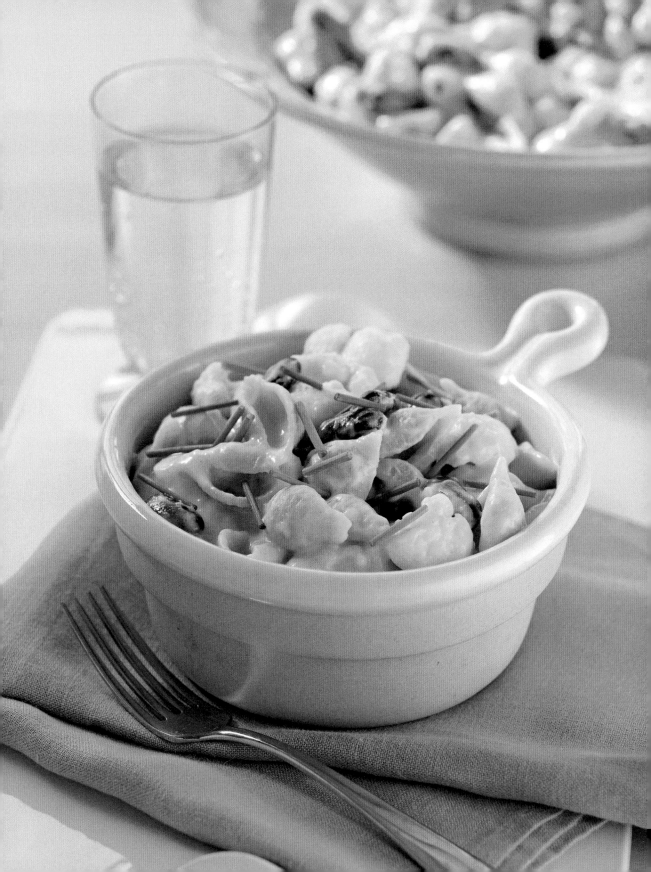

Tofu Cakes with Jícama Relish

MAKES 4 servings   HANDS-ON TIME: 10 minutes   TOTAL TIME: 25 minutes

If your block of tofu is less than 2 inches high, cut it horizontally in half (instead of into thirds) before cutting each piece crosswise in half for a total of 4 pieces instead of 12. If you like, make the tofu cakes and relish a day ahead and refrigerate separately. Both are delicious chilled or at room temperature.

14 to 16 ounces extra-firm tofu

6 tablespoons reduced-sodium soy sauce

5 tablespoons fresh lemon juice

2 teaspoons sesame oil

2 teaspoons grated lemon zest

Salt and freshly ground black pepper

½ pound jícama, peeled and finely diced

1 small red bell pepper, diced

3 scallions, minced

Heat the oven to 400°F. Cut the block of tofu horizontally into thirds. Cut each piece into quarters and place in a 9 × 9-inch baking pan.

In a small bowl, combine the soy sauce, 3 tablespoons of the lemon juice, and the sesame oil. Add to the tofu pieces, turning them to coat. Sprinkle the tops with the lemon zest and season lightly with salt and black pepper.

Bake for 20 minutes, or until the tofu is heated through.

Meanwhile, in a medium bowl, combine the jícama, bell pepper, scallions, and remaining 2 tablespoons lemon juice. Season with salt and black pepper to taste.

Divide the tofu evenly among 4 serving plates. Drizzle each serving with some sauce from the pan and serve with ½ cup jícama relish alongside.

NUTRITION AT A GLANCE

Per serving: 168 calories, 8 g fat, 1 g saturated fat, 12 g protein, 13 g carbohydrate, 2 g fiber, 872 mg sodium

Cook Once, Eat Twice

Double the recipe and refrigerate the extra tofu and jícama separately. The following day, recombine and serve cold or at room temperature.

Almond and Chickpea Burgers with Chipotle Mayo

MAKES 4 servings   **HANDS-ON TIME: 15 minutes**   **TOTAL TIME: 25 minutes**

The flavor of these veggie burgers is reminiscent of falafel but without all of the deep frying.

2 garlic cloves, unpeeled

½ cup slivered almonds (2 ounces)

1 can (19 ounces) chickpeas, drained and rinsed

¼ cup chopped fresh parsley

1 teaspoon ground cumin

½ teaspoon ground coriander

Pinch salt

1 large egg

4 teaspoons extra-virgin olive oil

2 tablespoons mayonnaise

½ teaspoon minced chipotle pepper in adobo, or to taste

4 (6-inch) whole-wheat pita breads

2 cups shredded Romaine lettuce

1 beefsteak tomato, coarsely chopped

In a small pan of boiling water, cook the garlic for 3 minutes to soften. When cool enough to handle, peel, transfer to a large bowl, and mash with a fork.

Meanwhile, in a small ungreased skillet over medium heat, toast the almonds for 3 to 5 minutes, until lightly browned and fragrant. Transfer to a mini food processor and pulse on and off to grind the almonds to a fine meal.

Add the chickpeas to the garlic and mash with a potato masher until no whole chickpeas remain. Add the almond meal, parsley, cumin, coriander, and salt. Stir to blend. Add the egg and mix well. Shape the mixture into 4 patties.

In a large nonstick skillet, heat the oil over medium heat. Add the patties and cook until browned and crisp on the outside and heated through, about 5 minutes per side.

Meanwhile, in a small bowl, blend the mayonnaise and chipotle pepper.

Spread each burger with 1½ teaspoons of the chipotle mayonnaise. For each pita, place one-eighth of the lettuce and tomato in the bottom part of the pita, add a burger, then top with another one-eighth of the lettuce and tomato.

NUTRITION AT A GLANCE
Per serving: 386 calories, 21 g fat, 2 g saturated fat, 17 g protein, 44 g carbohydrate, 16 g fiber, 465 mg sodium

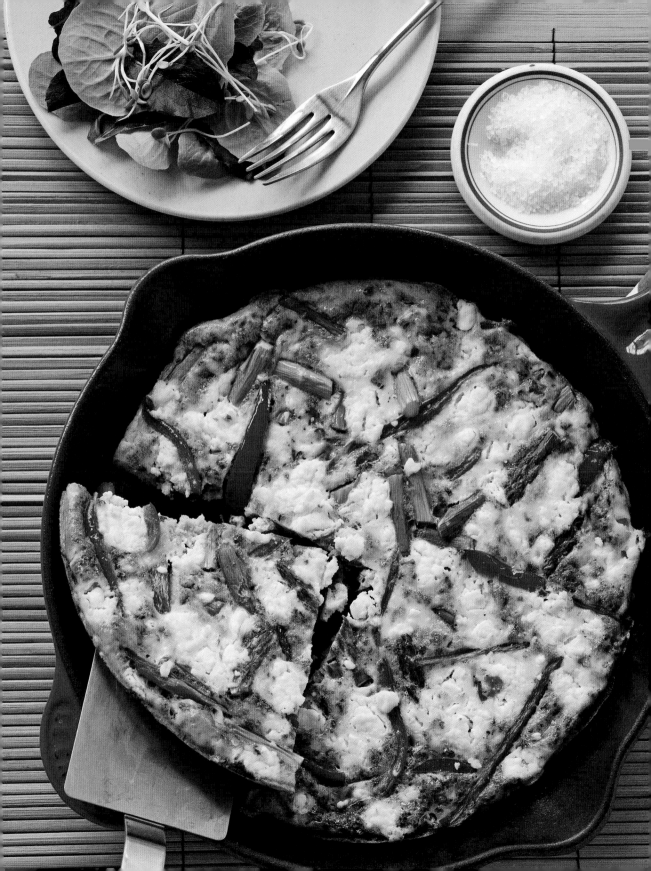

Asparagus and Red Pepper Frittata with Goat Cheese

MAKES 4 servings   HANDS-ON TIME: 10 minutes   TOTAL TIME: 30 minutes

One large wedge of this frittata makes a filling and healthy dinner, but you can easily serve the frittata in smaller pieces as a first course. If your nonstick pan has a plastic handle, wrap it in foil. It will be fine for the 3 minutes the pan is under the broiler.

- 3   teaspoons extra-virgin olive oil
- ½   pound asparagus, cut into ½-inch lengths
- 1   large red bell pepper, slivered
- 4   large eggs
- 3   large egg whites
- 1   teaspoon dried tarragon or Italian seasoning

- ¼   teaspoon salt
- ¼   teaspoon cracked black pepper
- 1   teaspoon trans-fat-free margarine (vegetable oil spread)
- 3   ounces reduced-fat goat cheese

In a 10-inch broilerproof nonstick skillet, heat 1 teaspoon of the oil over medium heat. Add the asparagus and bell pepper and cook, stirring, for 1 minute. Cover and cook for 2 minutes.

Meanwhile, in a medium bowl, whisk together the whole eggs, egg whites, tarragon, salt, and black pepper.

Reduce the heat to low and add the remaining 2 teaspoons oil and the margarine to the pan. Stir well to melt the margarine and to coat the bottom and sides of the pan with oil. Pour in the egg mixture and dot the top with the goat cheese. Cook, uncovered without stirring, until the eggs are set around the edge and still a little wet in the center, 12 to 14 minutes.

Meanwhile, heat the broiler.

Broil the frittata 6 inches from the heat for 2 to 3 minutes, until the top is just set and the cheese is melted. Cut into 4 wedges and serve hot, warm, at room temperature, or chilled.

NUTRITION AT A GLANCE
Per serving: 181 calories, 12 g fat, 3 g saturated fat, 14 g protein, 6 g carbohydrate, 2 g fiber, 343 mg sodium

Stir-Fried Seitan with Mushrooms and Leeks

MAKES 4 servings HANDS-ON TIME: 25 minutes TOTAL TIME: 25 minutes

Seitan, also called wheat gluten, is a delicious vegetarian protein. Look for it in health-food stores or in the produce section of your supermarket. It comes seasoned in a variety of ways, so choose your favorite.

- 2 teaspoons extra-virgin olive oil
- 1 medium red bell pepper, cut into 1-inch pieces
- 2 leeks, halved lengthwise, rinsed well, and cut into 1-inch lengths
- 8 ounces white mushrooms, quartered
- 2 garlic cloves, sliced
- 1 tablespoon minced fresh ginger

- ½ teaspoon salt
- 8 ounces seitan, cut into 1-inch chunks
- 2 tablespoons pine nuts
- 2 teaspoons rice vinegar
- 1 teaspoon dark sesame oil
- 4 cups shredded green cabbage

In a large nonstick skillet or wok, heat the oil over medium heat. Add the bell pepper, leeks, mushrooms, garlic, ginger, and salt. Cook, stirring frequently, until the vegetables are crisp-tender, 5 to 7 minutes.

Add the seitan to the pan and cook, stirring frequently, until heated through, about 3 minutes. Add the pine nuts, vinegar, and sesame oil and toss to combine.

Divide the cabbage among 4 plates, top with the stir-fry, and serve warm.

NUTRITION AT A GLANCE
Per serving: 431 calories, 8 g fat, 1 g saturated fat, 47 g protein, 36 g carbohydrate, 7 g fiber, 318 mg sodium

Variation: On Phase 2, have the stir-fry over ½ cup quick-cooking brown rice instead of cabbage.

Per serving (with brown rice): 464 calories, 8 g fat, 1 g saturated fat, 47 g protein, 43 g carbohydrate, 6 g fiber, 307 mg sodium

Vegetarian Black Bean Chili

MAKES 4 (1½-cup) servings **HANDS-ON TIME: 15 minutes** **TOTAL TIME: 25 minutes**

TVP stands for texturized vegetable protein. It's also sometimes called TSP, for texturized soy protein. Either is fine to use here. TVP is typically used to make vegetarian burgers and soy crumbles. If you can't find it, use the crumbles, or crumble up a veggie burger. Topping the chili with dairy-free soy yogurt keeps it vegan; nonvegans could use nonfat (0%) plain Greek yogurt instead.

- 4 teaspoons extra-virgin olive oil
- 2 medium red onions, coarsely chopped
- 6 garlic cloves, minced
- 1 teaspoon chipotle chile powder
- 1 teaspoon ground cumin
- ¾ cup TVP or TSP granules
- ¼ teaspoon salt

- 1 can (15.5 ounces) black beans, drained and rinsed
- 1 can (14.5 ounces) spicy diced tomatoes, with juice
- 1 can (8 ounces) no-salt-added tomato sauce
- 4 tablespoons nonfat plain soy yogurt

In a large nonstick skillet, heat the oil over medium heat. Add the onions, garlic, chipotle powder, and cumin. Cook, stirring often, until the onions begin to soften, about 3 minutes.

Stir in the TVP granules, salt, and 1½ cups water. Cook, stirring, for 1 minute to soften the TVP. Add the black beans, diced tomatoes and their juice, and tomato sauce. Simmer for 10 minutes to blend the flavors.

Divide the chili among 4 bowls and dollop each serving with 1 tablespoon yogurt.

NUTRITION AT A GLANCE
Per serving: 250 calories, 5 g fat, 1 g saturated fat, 16 g protein, 34 g carbohydrate, 10 g fiber, 695 mg sodium

Cook Once, Eat Twice

Double or triple the recipe and add enough vegetable broth to turn it into a hearty soup. Or, freeze what you aren't serving immediately, then reheat the frozen chili in the microwave, or thaw overnight in the fridge and reheat on the stovetop over low heat.

Acorn Squash and Two-Bean Gratin

MAKES 4 (2-cup) servings   HANDS-ON TIME: 15 minutes   TOTAL TIME: 30 minutes

In this delicious high-fiber vegetarian gratin, a topping of reduced-fat cheese and pumpkin seeds replaces the usual full-fat cheese and buttery bread crumbs.

1   small acorn squash (10 to 12 ounces)

1   can (15.5 ounces) black beans, drained and rinsed

1   can (15.5 ounces) pinto beans, drained and rinsed

2   tablespoons fresh lime juice

4   teaspoons extra-virgin olive oil

1½ teaspoons chili powder

1½ teaspoons ground coriander

1½ teaspoons dried oregano

¾   teaspoon salt

3   plum tomatoes, thinly sliced

1   cup shredded reduced-fat Mexican blend cheese (4 ounces)

¼   cup hulled pumpkin seeds

Heat the oven to 450°F. Bring a medium pot of water to a boil.

Meanwhile, halve the acorn squash lengthwise. Scoop out and discard the seeds and stringy strands. Thinly slice the squash crosswise, leaving the skin on.

Place the squash in the boiling water and cook until crisp-tender, about 3 minutes. Drain.

While the squash is cooking, in a large bowl, stir together the black beans, pinto beans, lime juice, oil, chili powder, coriander, oregano, and salt.

Add the drained squash and the tomatoes to the bean mixture and toss. Transfer to a 9 × 13-inch baking dish. Cover tightly with foil. Bake for 10 minutes, or until piping hot.

Uncover, top with the cheese and seeds, and bake for 5 minutes longer, or until the cheese has melted. Serve hot.

NUTRITION AT A GLANCE
Per serving: 326 calories, 15 g fat, 4 g saturated fat, 19 g protein, 34 g carbohydrate, 9 g fiber, 660 mg sodium

TIP: If you have cooked dried beans on hand, substitute 3½ cups total of one of your favorites for the canned beans in this recipe.

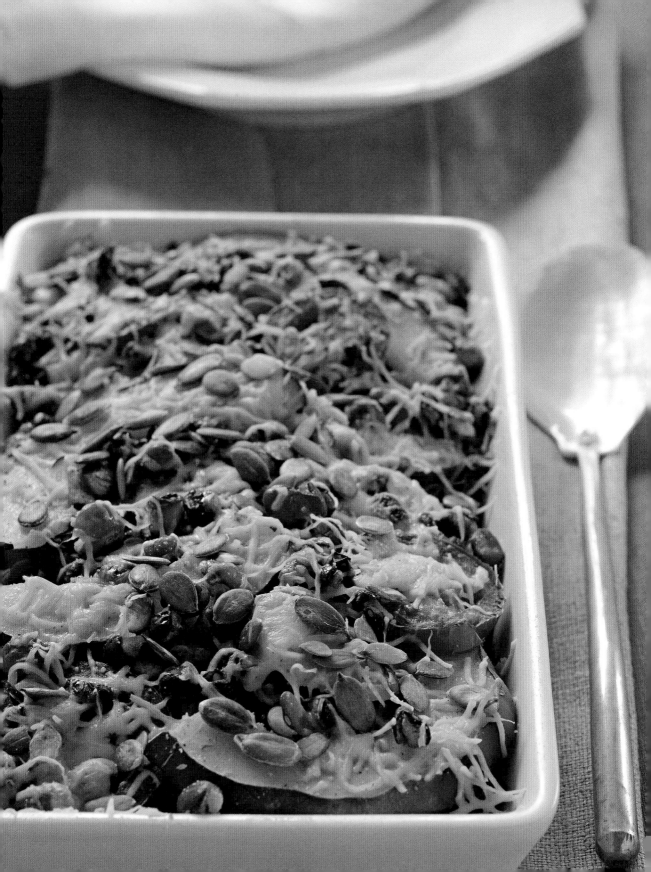

Picadillo-Style Lentil Stew

MAKES 4 (2-cup) servings   HANDS-ON TIME: 15 minutes   TOTAL TIME: 30 minutes

A picadillo is a salty-sweet Latin American dish typically made with beef, raisins, and olives. In this meatless Phase 1 version, we use a bell pepper instead of fruit.

1½ cups dried lentils, picked over and rinsed

4 garlic cloves, minced

¾ teaspoon salt

1 tablespoon extra-virgin olive oil

1 medium sweet onion, coarsely chopped

1 medium zucchini, coarsely diced

1 large red bell pepper, diced

1 can (15 ounces) no-salt-added tomato sauce

⅓ cup pimiento-stuffed green olives, sliced

1 tablespoon chili powder

2 teaspoons unsweetened cocoa powder, preferably dark

2 teaspoons granular sugar substitute

4 tablespoons nonfat (0%) plain Greek yogurt

Hot pepper sauce, for serving (optional)

In a medium saucepan, combine the lentils, garlic, salt, and 6 cups hot water. Bring to a boil over high heat. Reduce the heat and simmer, partially covered, for 15 to 20 minutes, until the lentils are just tender. Drain, reserving the cooking liquid.

While the lentils are cooking, in a large saucepan, heat the oil over medium heat. Add the onion and cook, stirring occasionally, until softened, about 5 minutes.

Stir in the zucchini and bell pepper. Cook for 1 minute longer. Add the tomato sauce, olives, chili powder, cocoa powder, and sugar substitute. Bring to a simmer and cook, stirring occasionally, until the zucchini and pepper are crisp-tender, about 10 minutes.

Add the lentils to the stew along with 1 cup of the reserved liquid. Simmer for 3 minutes to meld flavors. Serve topped with 1 tablespoon yogurt. Offer hot pepper sauce as an optional addition.

NUTRITION AT A GLANCE
Per serving: 354 calories, 6 g fat, 1 g saturated fat, 19 g protein, 59 g carbohydrate, 14 g fiber, 574 mg sodium

Cook Once, Eat Twice

Add vegetable broth to the stew and turn it into a soup. Or reheat and serve over whole-wheat pasta for Phase 2.

Thai Vegetable Stew

MAKES 4 (2¼-cup) servings   HANDS-ON TIME: 15 minutes   TOTAL TIME: 30 minutes

The flavors of coconut milk, basil, and lime give this stew its Thai overtones, but it's also fun to experiment with other ingredients. If you prefer yellow squash, use it instead of zucchini. Snow peas can stand in for the green beans (toss them in during the last minute of cooking). Try cilantro or mint instead of basil. Or use 1¾ cups of any canned or cooked dried beans you prefer.

4 teaspoons extra-virgin olive oil	1 (2-inch) piece fresh ginger, peeled and grated
1 small Italian eggplant, halved lengthwise and thinly sliced	½ teaspoon salt
1 small sweet potato, peeled, halved lengthwise, and thinly sliced	1 can (15.5 ounces) red beans, drained and rinsed
4 ounces white mushrooms, halved	1 package (about 14 ounces) medium-firm or firm tofu, drained, patted dry, and cut into 1-inch chunks
1 zucchini, halved lengthwise and thinly sliced	
4 ounces green beans, trimmed and halved crosswise (1 cup)	¾ cup unsweetened lite coconut milk
	½ cup fresh basil leaves, shredded
3 garlic cloves, slivered	2 tablespoons fresh lime juice

In a Dutch oven or large heavy-bottomed pot, heat the oil over medium heat. Add the eggplant and sweet potato and cook until the eggplant is beginning to brown, about 3 minutes.

Add the mushrooms, zucchini, green beans, garlic, ginger, salt, and ¾ cup water. Bring to a boil. Cook, uncovered, until the sweet potato is tender, about 7 minutes.

Stir in the red beans, tofu, and coconut milk. Cook until lightly thickened, about 3 minutes. Stir in the basil and lime juice. Divide the stew evenly among 4 bowls and serve hot.

NUTRITION AT A GLANCE
Per serving: 328 calories, 13 g fat, 3.5 g saturated fat, 18 g protein, 39 g carbohydrate, 13 g fiber, 547 mg sodium

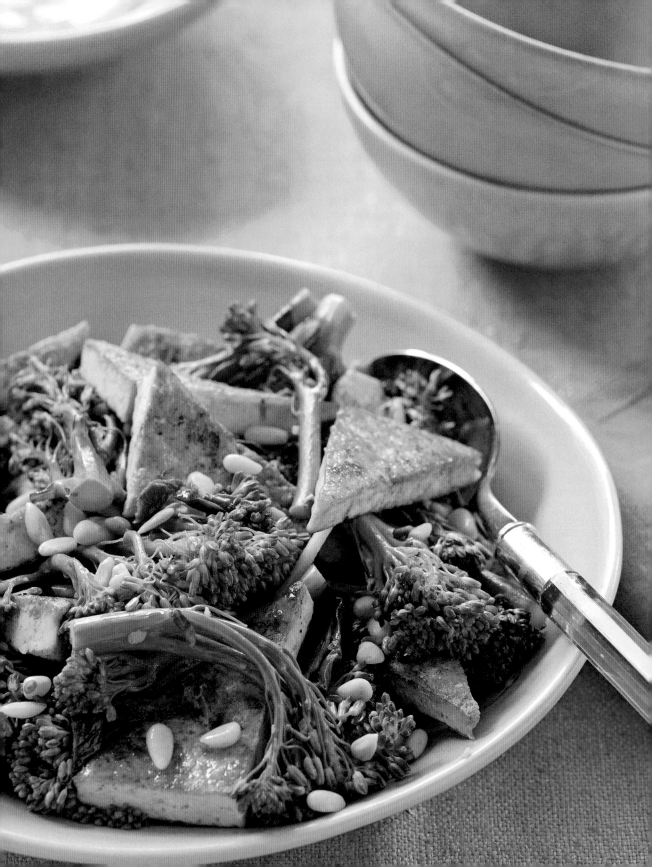

Crispy Tofu with Broccolini

MAKES 4 servings   **HANDS-ON TIME: 15 minutes**   **TOTAL TIME: 25 minutes**

Peanut oil brings extra flavor to this dish, but extra-virgin olive oil can be used instead. Don't be tempted to turn the tofu before it has developed a crust or it will stick to the pan. If broccolini (a cross between broccoli and Chinese kale) isn't available, use regular broccoli and cut it into thin florets, leaving some of the stems on.

- 1 pound medium-firm tofu, drained and patted dry
- ½ teaspoon five-spice powder
- ¾ teaspoon salt
- 1 tablespoon peanut oil
- 1 (12-ounce) head broccolini, trimmed
- ⅓ cup sun-dried tomato halves, thinly sliced
- 2 garlic cloves, slivered
- 1 (1-inch) piece fresh ginger, peeled and finely chopped
- ¼ cup pine nuts (1 ounce)

Cut the tofu into 6 slabs about 1 inch thick, then cut each diagonally in half to make 12 triangles. Sprinkle the tofu evenly with the five-spice powder and ½ teaspoon of the salt.

In a large nonstick skillet, heat the oil over medium heat. Add the tofu and cook, without turning, until a crust forms on the bottoms, about 3 minutes.

Using a wide spatula, turn the tofu over and cook until a crust forms on the other side, 3 to 4 minutes longer. With the spatula, transfer to a plate.

Add the broccolini and sun-dried tomatoes to the skillet and cook, tossing, for 1 minute. Add the garlic, ginger, remaining ¼ teaspoon salt, and ½ cup water. Cover and cook until the broccolini is crisp-tender, 3 to 4 minutes.

Add the pine nuts and toss. Transfer the broccoli mixture to a platter and mix gently with the tofu. Serve warm.

NUTRITION AT A GLANCE
Per serving: 208 calories, 13 g fat, 2 g saturated fat, 14 g protein, 12 g carbohydrate, 3 g fiber, 570 mg sodium

Herbed Quinoa and Edamame

MAKES 4 (1½-cup) servings   HANDS-ON TIME: 10 minutes   TOTAL TIME: 30 minutes

We recommend keeping edamame on hand in the freezer for quick protein-packed meatless meals. It is available in your supermarket's freezer section both shelled and unshelled (use shelled for this recipe).

2	teaspoons extra-virgin olive oil	2	cups frozen shelled edamame
3	scallions, thinly sliced	4	cups baby spinach
2	garlic cloves, slivered	½	cup whole fresh parsley leaves
1	cup quinoa, rinsed and drained	¼	cup fresh mint, chopped
1½	teaspoons grated lime zest	2	teaspoons trans-fat-free margarine (vegetable oil spread)
¾	teaspoon salt		

In a large saucepan, heat the oil over medium heat. Add the scallions and garlic and cook until the scallions wilt, about 1 minute.

Add the quinoa, lime zest, salt, and 1½ cups water. Bring to a boil. Reduce the heat to a simmer, cover, and cook for 7 minutes.

Add the edamame, cover, and cook for about 5 minutes longer, until the quinoa has absorbed the liquid and the edamame are tender.

Add the spinach, parsley, mint, and margarine and stir to combine. Serve warm.

NUTRITION AT A GLANCE
Per serving: 313 calories, 10 g fat, 1 g saturated fat, 15 g protein, 41 g carbohydrate, 9 g fiber, 530 mg sodium

Cook Once, Eat Twice

Double the recipe and add cooked chicken or turkey, a little lemon juice, and some extra-virgin olive oil for a salad.

African Red Bean Stew

MAKES 4 (1½-cup) servings   HANDS-ON TIME: 15 minutes   TOTAL TIME: 30 minutes

Okra is a traditional addition to many stews, including African specialties. If you're not a fan of this vegetable, substitute frozen broccoli.

2 teaspoons extra-virgin olive oil

1 medium onion, finely chopped

1 medium green bell pepper, cut into ½-inch dice

2 garlic cloves, thinly sliced

¼ teaspoon dried thyme

3 tablespoons tomato paste

¾ teaspoon salt

2 cans (15.5 ounces each) no-salt-added pinto beans, drained and rinsed

1 package (10 ounces) frozen sliced okra

1 cup lower-sodium chicken or vegetable broth

2 tablespoons natural no-sugar-added creamy peanut butter

⅛ teaspoon cayenne pepper

In a Dutch oven or large pot, heat the oil over medium heat. Add the onion, bell pepper, garlic, and thyme. Cook, stirring occasionally, until the vegetables are tender, about 7 minutes.

Stir in the tomato paste and salt. Cook for 1 minute. Stir in the beans, okra, and broth. Bring to a boil, then reduce the heat to a simmer. Cover and cook for 5 minutes, or until the okra is tender.

Whisk in the peanut butter and cayenne and simmer for 1 minute longer. Serve warm.

NUTRITION AT A GLANCE

Per serving: 253 calories, 7 g fat, 1 g saturated fat, 12 g protein, 36 g carbohydrate, 11 g fiber, 516 mg sodium

Variation: For a Phase 2 option, ladle the stew over ½ cup quick-cooking brown rice.

Per serving (with brown rice): 303 calories, 7 g fat, 1 g saturated fat, 14 g protein, 47 g carbohydrate, 12 g fiber, 517 mg sodium

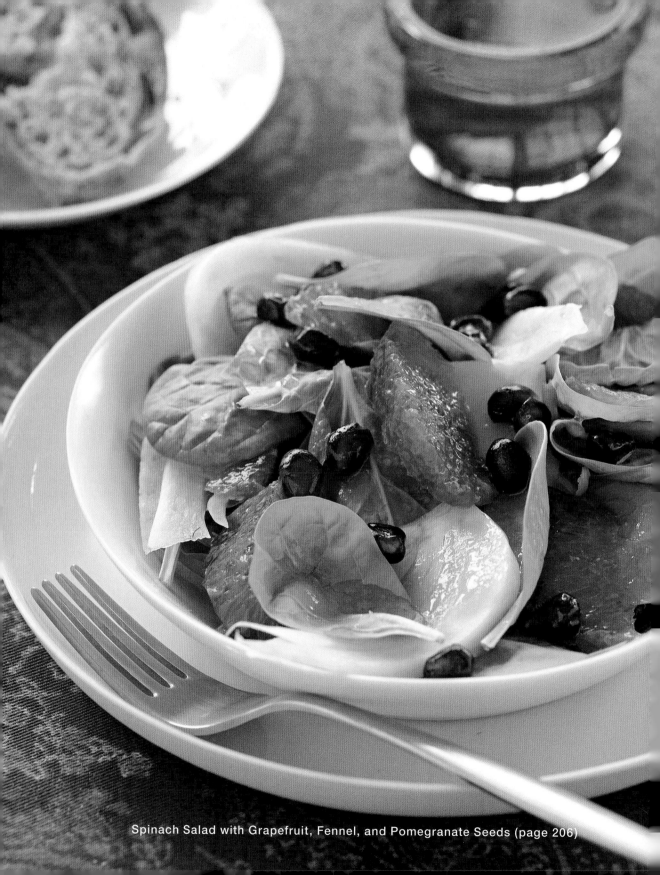

Spinach Salad with Grapefruit, Fennel, and Pomegranate Seeds (page 206)

SIDE DISHES, SIDE SALADS, AND SAUCES

It's one thing to cook a main course in a hurry, but don't forget the side salads, vegetable dishes, salsas, and special sauces that round out a meal and add essential nutrients as well. Whatever phase of the diet you're on, we recommend eating at least 2 cups of vegetables with lunch and dinner (and even at breakfast if you can work them in). And, of course, high-fiber sides made with whole grains like quinoa and barley are always on our recipe list to enjoy after Phase 1.

When you're shopping for produce, whether it's arugula, spinach, pears, or mangoes, buy what looks freshest in your market and adapt your side dishes accordingly. The Meal Plans on pages 268 to 297 will give you plenty of ideas for matching sides, salads, and sauces with the various meat, poultry, seafood, and meatless main dishes in this book.

Spinach Salad with Grapefruit, Fennel, and Pomegranate Seeds

MAKES 4 servings   HANDS-ON TIME: 25 minutes   TOTAL TIME: 25 minutes

A contrasting blend of flavors and colors makes this a spectacular salad for a festive lunch or dinner. Pomegranate seeds add a pleasant tart crunch, not to mention a healthy dose of antioxidants, including vitamin C. See the tip for how to neatly seed a pomegranate.

- 1 small fennel bulb, stalks trimmed off and outer skin removed
- 2 medium pink grapefruits
- 1 tablespoon sherry vinegar
- ½ teaspoon Dijon mustard
- ¼ cup extra-virgin olive oil
- Salt and freshly ground black pepper
- 1 package (5 ounces) baby spinach leaves
- ½ cup pomegranate seeds

Cut out and discard the core of the fennel bulb, then slice the bulb lengthwise into very thin strips; place in a serving bowl.

With a sharp paring knife, remove the peel and pith from the grapefruits. Working over a strainer set in a bowl, cut between the membranes to release the sections. Discard the membranes. Reserve 1 tablespoon of the grapefruit juice (squeeze the sections if you need more juice).

In a cup, combine the reserved 1 tablespoon juice, the vinegar, and mustard. Slowly whisk in the oil. Season with salt and pepper.

Add the grapefruit sections, spinach, and pomegranate seeds to the fennel. Drizzle with the dressing and toss to combine.

NUTRITION AT A GLANCE
Per serving: 204 calories, 14 g fat, 2 g saturated fat, 2 g protein, 20 g carbohydrate, 5 g fiber, 87 mg sodium

TIP: To remove the seeds from a pomegranate without covering yourself in juice, cut off the stem end, then score the fruit in 4 places. Submerge the scored fruit in a large bowl of cold water, then gently pull the sections apart. The seeds will sink to the bottom, the membranes will float to the top, and your hands and clothes will remain clean. Leftover seeds make a healthy snack or can be frozen in an airtight container for 3 months.

Shiitake Barley Pilaf

MAKES 4 (generous ½-cup) servings **HANDS-ON TIME: 10 minutes** **TOTAL TIME: 30 minutes**

This pilaf is made with quick-cooking barley that has been presteamed to cut the cooking time from the usual 45 minutes to about 10. To make this a main course, simply add cooked diced chicken or turkey breast along with some sliced almonds.

- 1 tablespoon extra-virgin olive oil
- 6 ounces fresh shiitake mushrooms, stems discarded, caps thinly sliced crosswise
- 2 garlic cloves, minced
- 1¾ cups lower-sodium chicken broth
- 1 cup quick-cooking barley
- 2 teaspoons grated lemon zest
- Salt and freshly ground black pepper
- ⅓ cup chopped fresh parsley

In a medium saucepan, heat the oil over medium heat. Add the shiitakes and garlic. Cook, stirring, until the shiitakes soften, about 2 minutes.

Add the broth, stirring to scrape up any browned bits, and bring to a boil over high heat. Add the barley, lemon zest, and salt and pepper to taste. Reduce the heat to a simmer, cover, and cook for 10 to 12 minutes, until the barley is tender.

Remove the pan from the heat and let stand for 5 minutes.

Stir in the parsley and serve warm.

NUTRITION AT A GLANCE
Per serving: 197 calories, 5 g fat, 1 g saturated fat, 7 g protein, 36 g carbohydrate, 5 g fiber, 36 mg sodium

Cook Once, Eat Twice

Double the recipe. The following day, add a little more olive oil to the extra, along with some lemon juice, thinly sliced scallions, and lean cooked ground beef for a hearty main-dish salad.

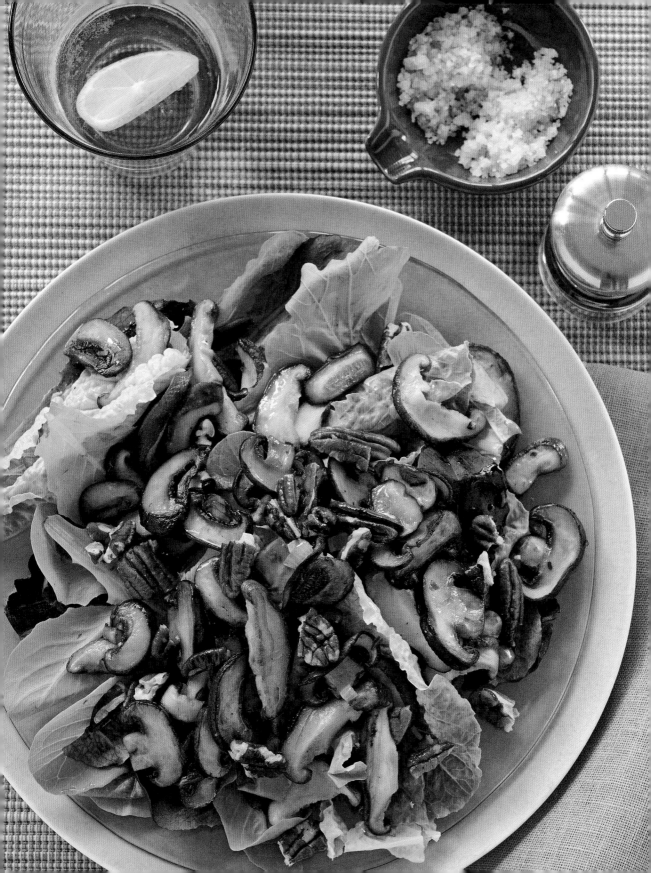

Warm Mushroom Salad with Toasted Pecans

MAKES 4 servings   **HANDS-ON TIME:** 15 minutes   **TOTAL TIME:** 15 minutes

Using both cremini and shiitake mushrooms gives more depth of flavor to this salad than white button mushrooms would (but you can use them, if you prefer). The warm mushrooms alone make a fine topper for the Satay Chicken Burgers, page 152.

2 large garlic cloves, minced

1 small shallot, minced

¼ teaspoon dried thyme

1 tablespoon plus 4 teaspoons extra-virgin olive oil

½ pound cremini mushrooms, sliced

½ pound fresh shiitake mushrooms, stems discarded, caps sliced

Salt and freshly ground black pepper

1 ounce pecan halves (¼ cup)

2 teaspoons balsamic vinegar

5 ounces mixed greens (about 8 cups)

In a large bowl, combine the garlic, shallot, thyme, and 1 tablespoon of the oil. Add the mushrooms and toss to coat.

In a large nonstick skillet, heat 2 teaspoons of the remaining oil over medium heat. Scrape in the mushroom mixture and cook, stirring often, until the mushrooms are just tender, about 5 minutes. Remove the pan from the heat and season the mushrooms with salt and pepper to taste.

While the mushrooms are cooking, toast the pecans in a 350°F toaster oven or in an ungreased skillet over medium heat for 3 to 5 minutes, until just beginning to brown (be careful, they burn quickly). Pour onto a cutting board to stop the cooking, then coarsely chop.

In the bowl that held the mushrooms, combine the remaining 2 teaspoons oil and the vinegar. Add the mixed greens and toss to coat.

Line 4 salad plates with the mixed greens and spoon the warm mushroom mixture on top. Sprinkle with the toasted pecans.

NUTRITION AT A GLANCE
Per serving: 181 calories, 14 g fat, 2 g saturated fat, 4 g protein, 14 g carbohydrate, 3 g fiber, 16 mg sodium

Braised Balsamic Carrots

MAKES 4 (1-cup) servings　**HANDS-ON TIME: 5 minutes**　**TOTAL TIME: 25 minutes**

Make a double batch of these carrots: They're delicious chilled and are a great grab-and-go snack that's tastier than plain baby carrots from a bag.

2　medium shallots or ½ small red onion, minced

1　tablespoon extra-virgin olive oil

1½　pounds baby carrots

2　tablespoons balsamic vinegar

Freshly ground black pepper

2　teaspoons granular sugar substitute

Salt

2　tablespoons chopped fresh chives (optional)

In a large nonstick saucepan, combine the shallots and oil. Add the carrots, vinegar, pepper to taste, and ⅓ cup water. Bring to a boil over medium-high heat. Reduce the heat to medium, cover, and cook for 20 minutes.

Uncover the pan, stir in the sugar substitute, and cook until the liquid has evaporated, about 3 minutes. Remove the pan from the heat, cover, and let sit for 2 minutes.

Season with salt to taste and stir in the chives (if using). Serve warm.

NUTRITION AT A GLANCE
Per serving: 109 calories, 4 g fat, 0.5 g saturated fat, 2 g protein, 18 g carbohydrate, 5 g fiber, 135 mg sodium

Roasted Green and Wax Beans with Walnuts

MAKES 4 servings   **HANDS-ON TIME: 10 minutes**   **TOTAL TIME: 25 minutes**

Mixing yellow and green beans enhances the flavor of this simple side dish. The beans are briefly blanched to preserve their color before roasting. Using both walnut oil and walnuts provides a double dose of heart-healthy omega-3 fatty acids.

½ pound green beans, trimmed

½ pound yellow wax beans, trimmed

2 tablespoons walnut oil

Salt and freshly ground black pepper

2 tablespoons coarsely chopped walnuts

Heat the oven to 350°F.

Bring a medium saucepan of water to a boil over high heat. Add the green beans and wax beans and return to a boil. Cook for 2 minutes. Transfer to a colander and rinse under cold water to stop the cooking. Drain again and pat dry.

Place the beans in 9 × 13-inch baking pan. Drizzle with the walnut oil and sprinkle lightly with salt and pepper to taste. Toss to coat. Add the walnuts and toss again. Roast the beans for 8 to 10 minutes, until tender and lightly browned in spots. Serve warm.

NUTRITION AT A GLANCE
Per serving: 115 calories, 9 g fat, 1 g saturated fat, 2 g protein, 8 g carbohydrate, 4 g fiber, 3 mg sodium

---

TIP: Walnut oil has a shelf life of about 3 months. Once opened, it should be kept in a cool dark place or refrigerated to prevent it from becoming rancid.

Cook Once, Eat Twice
Prepare a double batch and toss the extra with lemon juice or red wine vinegar for a salad.

Grilled Asparagus with Orange-Cumin Vinaigrette

MAKES 4 servings   HANDS-ON TIME: 15 minutes   TOTAL TIME: 25 minutes

Grilling lends a lightly caramelized taste to asparagus, while a drizzle of orange-cumin dressing provides a tangy flavor contrast. If you're grilling outdoors, use a grill topper to ensure that the spears don't fall through the grate. This recipe makes extra dressing, which you can keep in the fridge for up to a week or so and use on salads or other grilled vegetables.

1   bunch asparagus spears, trimmed (about 1 pound)

2   teaspoons plus ½ cup extra-virgin olive oil

Salt and freshly ground black pepper

1   teaspoon slivered or grated orange zest

⅓   cup fresh orange juice

3   tablespoons fresh lime juice

1   tablespoon minced red onion

1   large garlic clove, minced

2   teaspoons Dijon mustard

Generous pinch ground cumin

Heat a grill or grill pan to medium. Lay the asparagus in a single layer on a rimmed baking sheet. Drizzle with 2 teaspoons of the oil; season with salt and pepper and roll the spears to coat.

Grill the asparagus, turning at least once, until lightly browned, 5 to 8 minutes, depending on thickness (do not overcook). Transfer to a serving platter.

In a small bowl, whisk together the orange zest and juice, lime juice, onion, garlic, mustard, and cumin. Slowly whisk in the remaining ½ cup oil. Season with salt and pepper to taste.

Drizzle ¼ cup of the dressing over the asparagus and serve warm.

NUTRITION AT A GLANCE
Per serving: 111 calories, 10 g fat, 1 g saturated fat, 3 g protein, 5 g carbohydrate, 2 g fiber, 17 mg sodium

Variation: To make this a Phase 1 dish, substitute a prepared no-sugar-added dressing of your choice, such as balsamic vinaigrette, for the orange-cumin vinaigrette.

Per serving (with prepared balsamic vinaigrette): 84 calories, 6 g fat, 0.4 g saturated fat, 2 g protein, 6 g carbohydrate, 2 g fiber, 117 mg sodium

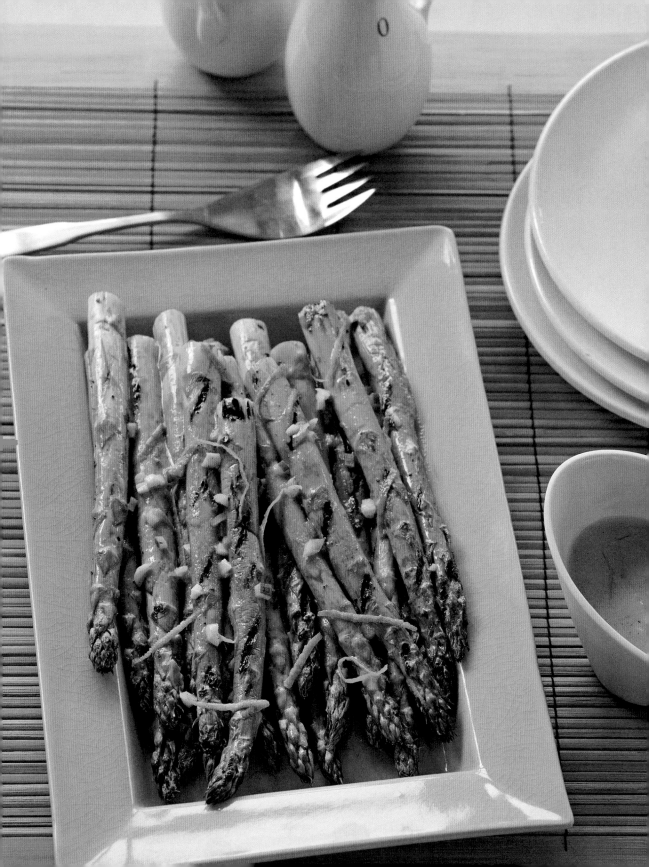

Summer Salad with Fresh Herb Vinaigrette

MAKES 4 servings   HANDS-ON TIME: 15 minutes   TOTAL TIME: 25 minutes

This side salad is a celebration of the garden-fresh vegetables and herbs of summer. Feel free to add other Phase 1 summer veggies, such as tomatoes and zucchini. If you don't like raw garlic in a salad, blanch the clove in the boiling water for about a minute before chopping.

½ pound green beans, halved

¼ pound sugar snap peas, strings removed

1 tablespoon finely chopped fresh basil, thyme, marjoram, chervil, or a combination

1 tablespoon finely chopped fresh parsley

1 tablespoon minced red onion

2 teaspoons sherry vinegar or other red wine vinegar

1 teaspoon Dijon mustard

1 garlic clove, minced

2 tablespoons extra-virgin olive oil

Salt and freshly ground black pepper

4 cups lightly packed baby lettuce leaves (about 3 ounces)

1 small cucumber, peeled, halved, seeded, and thinly sliced

1 small red bell pepper, diced

Bring a medium saucepan of lightly salted water to a boil over high heat. Add the green beans, return to a boil, and cook for 2 minutes. Using a slotted spoon or skimmer, transfer the beans to a colander and rinse under cold water to stop the cooking. Transfer to a plate.

Add the snap peas to the boiling water and cook for 30 seconds. Drain and rinse under cold water to stop the cooking. Halve the snap peas lengthwise. Pat the beans and snap peas dry.

In a cup, whisk together the basil (and/or other herbs), parsley, onion, vinegar, mustard, and garlic. Drizzle in the olive oil and whisk to combine. Season with salt and pepper to taste.

In a large serving bowl combine the beans, snap peas, lettuce, cucumber, and bell pepper. Pour the dressing over the salad and toss to coat.

NUTRITION AT A GLANCE
Per serving: 113 calories, 7 g fat, 1 g saturated fat, 3 g protein, 10 g carbohydrate, 5 g fiber, 50 mg sodium

Quick Creamed Spinach

MAKES 4 servings   HANDS-ON TIME: 20 minutes   TOTAL TIME: 20 minutes

Using frozen spinach cuts down on the prep time of this classic dish. You can easily double or triple the recipe for a big holiday or family dinner.

- 1 bag (16 ounces) frozen spinach, thawed
- ¾ cup fat-free milk
- 4 ounces reduced-fat cream cheese, cut into chunks and softened
- 2 teaspoons extra-virgin olive oil
- 1 small onion, minced
- Pinch ground nutmeg
- Salt and freshly ground black pepper
- ¼ cup grated Parmesan cheese (1 ounce)

Place the thawed spinach in a colander set over a large bowl; squeeze to extract the juice. Pour 2 tablespoons of the juice into a cup and reserve. Discard any remaining juice.

In a medium saucepan, combine the spinach juice, milk, and cream cheese. Bring to a simmer over low heat, stirring and pushing the cheese against the pan to break up. (The mixture should be well combined but will not be smooth.) Remove the pan from the heat.

In a large nonstick skillet, heat the oil over medium-low heat. Add the onion and cook, stirring frequently, until softened, about 3 minutes.

Add the spinach, stirring to coat. Stir in the milk mixture and cook until bubbling, about 3 minutes.

Season the spinach with nutmeg and salt and pepper to taste. Sprinkle with the Parmesan and serve hot.

NUTRITION AT A GLANCE
Per serving: 152 calories, 9 g fat, 4 g saturated fat, 10 g protein, 11 g carbohydrate, 4 g fiber, 313 mg sodium

TIP: When shopping for frozen spinach for this recipe, make sure to select a brand without added butter sauce.

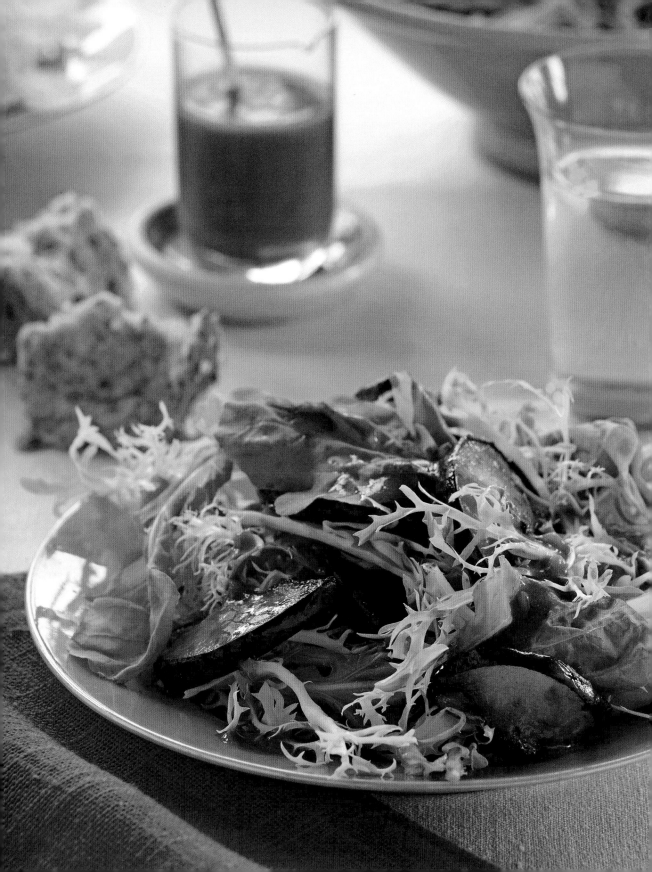

Arugula, Frisée, and Roasted Pear Salad

MAKES 4 servings   HANDS-ON TIME: 15 minutes   TOTAL TIME: 25 minutes

Mellow roasted pears are the perfect flavor contrast to peppery arugula and spicy frisée. The amount of vinaigrette here is more than you will need for the salad. Just keep the extra in the fridge and use it on other salads or as a marinade for chicken or turkey.

2 red Bartlett pears, skin left on

1 tablespoon plus ½ cup extra-virgin olive oil

3 tablespoons balsamic vinegar

1 tablespoon Dijon mustard

1 small garlic clove, minced

1 teaspoon minced onion or shallot

Pinch dried thyme

1 package (about 7 ounces) prewashed arugula

1 small head frisée, leaves torn into bite-size pieces

Heat the oven to 450°F. Line a baking sheet with foil.

Meanwhile, halve, core, and slice the pears crosswise into 8 slices each. Place in a small bowl, sprinkle with 1 tablespoon of the oil, and toss to coat well.

Place the pears on the baking sheet and roast, turning once halfway through cooking, for 10 minutes.

Meanwhile, in a cup, whisk together the vinegar, mustard, garlic, onion, and thyme. Slowly whisk in the remaining ½ cup oil.

In a large serving bowl, toss the arugula and frisée with ¼ cup of the vinaigrette. Add the roasted pears, tossing to coat. Serve while the pears are still warm.

NUTRITION AT A GLANCE

Per serving: 190 calories, 13 g fat, 2 g saturated fat, 2 g protein, 18 g carbohydrate, 5 g fiber, 53 mg sodium

TIP: If you can't find packaged prewashed arugula, buy two heads and give them a good wash. If frisée is unavailable, substitute watercress or baby spinach.

Indian-Spiced Mashed Sweet Potatoes

MAKES 4 (¾-cup) servings   HANDS-ON TIME: 10 minutes   TOTAL TIME: 20 minutes

Sweet potatoes—an outstanding source of carotenoids (including beta-carotene), vitamin C, calcium, and potassium—are one of our favorite South Beach Diet foods and a healthy alternative to white potatoes. They can vary widely in texture; some are wet when cooked and others are a little dry. If you find these potatoes dry after mashing, add a little water to help smooth them out.

1¼ pounds (about 4 medium) sweet potatoes, peeled and cut into 1-inch chunks

1 teaspoon garam masala

½ teaspoon salt

½ teaspoon ground cumin

½ teaspoon ground ginger

4 teaspoons extra-virgin olive oil

2 teaspoons fresh lime juice

In a steamer, cook the sweet potatoes for 10 to 15 minutes, until tender when pierced with the tip of a knife.

Transfer to a large bowl and add the garam masala, salt, cumin, and ginger. Mash with a potato masher (or use an immersion blender) to combine. Add the oil and lime juice and mash again.

NUTRITION AT A GLANCE
Per serving: 132 calories, 5 g fat, 1 g saturated fat, 2 g protein, 21 g carbohydrate, 4 g fiber, 357 mg sodium

TIP: Look for garam masala in Indian markets or in the spice section of your supermarket. See page 102 for more on this spice blend.

Cook Once, Eat Twice

Prepare a double batch and add some fat-free evaporated milk and lower-sodium chicken broth to the extra to make a soup. Garnish with chopped scallions, if desired.

Fennel, Cucumber, and Watercress Salad

15 MINUTE RECIPE

MAKES 4 servings   **HANDS-ON TIME: 10 minutes**   **TOTAL TIME: 10 minutes**

This year-round salad lends a refreshing element to any meal. Fennel has a mild, anise-like flavor that complements the peppery watercress. Serve the salad with Inside-Out Cheeseburgers, page 147.

1   small fennel bulb (about 8 ounces), stalks trimmed off and outer skin removed

½   medium cucumber, peeled

2   tablespoons fresh lemon juice

1   tablespoon extra-virgin olive oil

1   medium bunch watercress, tough ends trimmed

2   tablespoons minced red onion

Salt and freshly ground black pepper

Quarter the fennel bulb lengthwise and remove the hard core. Thinly slice the quarters crosswise. Halve the cucumber lengthwise, then slice into thin half-moons.

In a medium serving bowl, whisk together the lemon juice and oil.

Add the fennel, cucumber, watercress, and onion to the dressing and toss to coat. Season with salt and pepper to taste.

NUTRITION AT A GLANCE
Per serving: 58 calories, 4 g fat, 0.5 g saturated fat, 1 g protein, 6 g carbohydrate, 2 g fiber, 36 mg sodium

Lemon Quinoa Salad

MAKES 4 servings   HANDS-ON TIME: 10 minutes   TOTAL TIME: 30 minutes

Quinoa is sometimes called a "supergrain" because it contains both fiber and protein. It also has a mild nutty flavor, making it a tasty alternative to brown rice. This lemon-infused salad makes a perfect partner for Flank Steak with Chimichurri, page 175.

¾ cup quinoa

Salt

2 tablespoons fresh lemon juice

1 tablespoon extra-virgin olive oil

2 celery stalks with leaves, thinly sliced

1 medium red bell pepper, diced

¼ cup thinly sliced basil leaves

Freshly ground black pepper

¼ cup slivered almonds

Place the quinoa in a strainer and rinse under cold running water for 2 minutes.

In a medium saucepan, bring 1¾ cups lightly salted water to a boil over high heat. Stir in the quinoa and reduce the heat to low. Cover and simmer for 15 to 20 minutes, until the water is absorbed. Remove the pan from the heat and let stand for 5 minutes.

Meanwhile, make the dressing: In a small bowl, whisk together the lemon juice and oil.

In a large bowl, combine the quinoa, celery, bell pepper, and basil. Add the dressing and toss well. Season with salt and pepper to taste. Sprinkle the salad with the slivered almonds and serve warm or at room temperature.

NUTRITION AT A GLANCE
Per serving: 203 calories, 9 g fat, 1 g saturated fat, 6 g protein, 25 g carbohydrate, 4 g fiber, 19 mg sodium

TIPS: Don't skip the rinsing of the quinoa. The grains have a natural coating called saponin, which gives the quinoa a bitter flavor if not rinsed off. For a quick way to thinly slice basil, see the tip on page 186.

Cook Once, Eat Twice

Make a double batch. Cut pockets in bone-in chicken breasts, stuff with the salad, then roast.

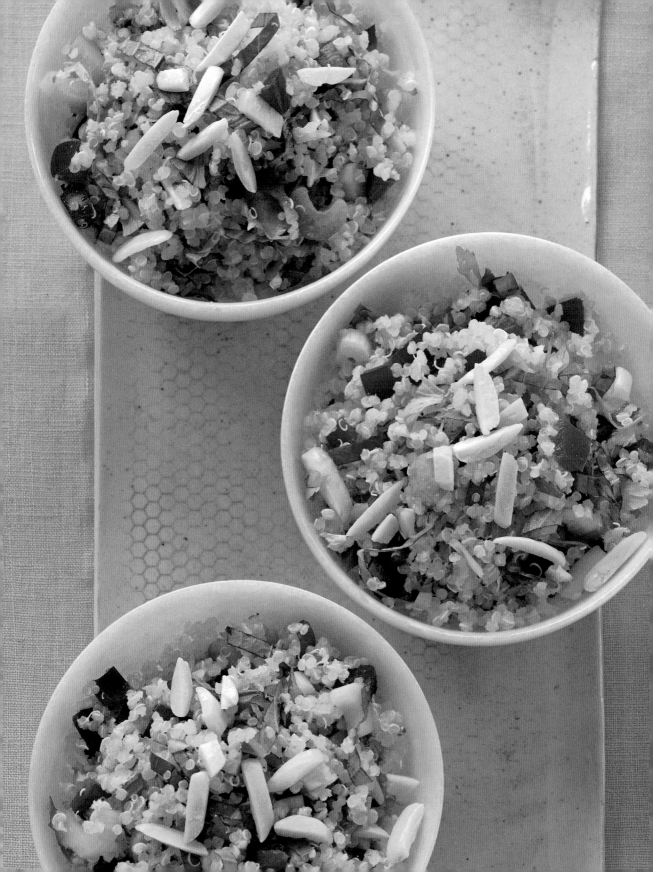

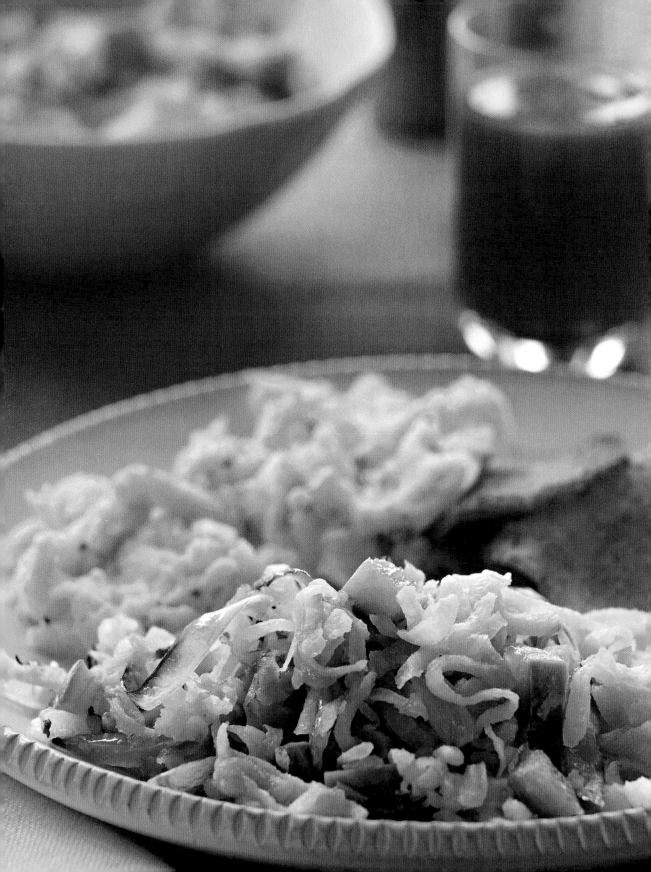

Jícama Hash Browns

MAKES 4 (½-cup) servings   HANDS-ON TIME: 20 minutes   TOTAL TIME: 20 minutes

Phase 1 dieters will love this nonstarchy alternative to potatoes for breakfast or anytime. The hash browns are a great side for grilled steak or chicken. For info on jícama, see page 80.

- 2 tablespoons extra-virgin olive oil
- 1 medium onion, thinly sliced
- 1 medium green bell pepper, diced
- 1 medium jícama (12 ounces)

- ½ teaspoon salt
- ¼ teaspoon freshly ground black pepper

In a large nonstick skillet, heat the oil over medium heat. Add the onion and bell pepper and cook, stirring frequently, until the vegetables are tender, about 7 minutes.

Meanwhile, peel the jícama, then shred on the large holes of a box grater.

Add the jícama to the pan with the vegetables and cook, stirring, for 1 minute. Add ¼ cup water, the salt, and the black pepper. Cook, stirring frequently, until the jícama begins to brown and is crisp-tender, about 7 minutes. Serve warm.

NUTRITION AT A GLANCE
Per serving: 112 calories, 7 g fat, 1 g saturated fat, 1 g protein, 12 g carbohydrate, 1 g fiber, 296 mg sodium

Baby Greens and Grilled Asparagus with Shallot Vinaigrette

MAKES 4 servings   HANDS-ON TIME: 15 minutes   TOTAL TIME: 20 minutes

For this side salad, use the freshest baby greens you can find at your supermarket or farmers' market. The garnish of toasted pumpkin seeds provides vitamin E, magnesium, and zinc. You can also purchase the pumpkin seeds already roasted if you prefer.

- 2 tablespoons hulled pumpkin seeds
- 2 tablespoons fresh lemon juice
- 2 teaspoons balsamic vinegar
- 1 large shallot, minced
- 1 teaspoon Dijon mustard
- Salt and freshly ground black pepper

- 2 tablespoons extra-virgin olive oil
- 1 small bunch slender asparagus (about 12 ounces)
- 5 cups baby salad greens (about 4 ounces)

Heat a grill or grill pan to medium.

In a small ungreased skillet, toast the pumpkin seeds over medium heat until they look lightly browned and puffed up a bit, 3 to 5 minutes. Scrape onto a plate to stop the cooking.

In a cup, combine the lemon juice, vinegar, shallot, mustard, and salt and pepper to taste. Whisk in the oil until well blended.

Place the asparagus in a shallow bowl. Drizzle with 2 tablespoons of the vinaigrette and turn the spears to coat.

Grill the asparagus, turning often, until lightly browned, 3 to 5 minutes, depending on thickness. Transfer to a cutting board and cut on the diagonal into 1-inch pieces.

In a large bowl, toss the asparagus and greens with the remaining dressing. Divide the salad among 4 plates and sprinkle each serving evenly with pumpkin seeds.

NUTRITION AT A GLANCE

Per serving: 115 calories, 9 g fat, 1 g saturated fat, 4 g protein, 7 g carbohydrate, 3 g fiber, 41 mg sodium

Chickpea and Edamame Salad

MAKES 4 servings   HANDS-ON TIME: 15 minutes   TOTAL TIME: 25 minutes

Both chickpeas and edamame are high in appetite-satisfying fiber. In fact, just the 1 cup of shelled edamame in this healthy salad contributes a whopping 6 grams of fiber to each serving.

1 tablespoon extra-virgin olive oil

½ teaspoon grated lemon zest

2 tablespoons fresh lemon juice

1 garlic clove, minced

1 tablespoon chopped fresh mint

  Salt and freshly ground black pepper

1 can (15 ounces) chickpeas, drained and rinsed

1 cup frozen shelled edamame, thawed

3 radishes, thinly sliced

½ small red onion, very thinly sliced

In a large serving bowl, combine the oil, lemon zest, lemon juice, garlic, mint, and salt and pepper to taste. Add the chickpeas and toss to coat.

Bring a small saucepan of salted water to a boil. Add the edamame and cook until heated through, about 4 minutes. Drain and rinse under cold water. Drain again and pat dry.

Add the edamame, radishes, and onion to the bowl with the chickpeas and toss well.

NUTRITION AT A GLANCE
Per serving: 181 calories, 6 g fat, 0.6 g saturated fat, 8 g protein, 24 g carbohydrate, 6 g fiber, 248 mg sodium

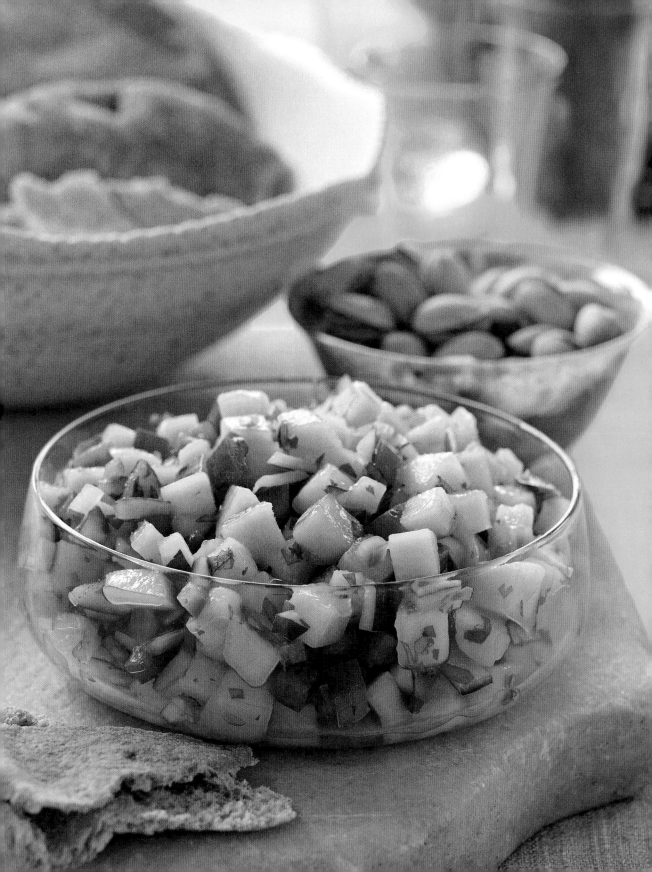

Mango Salsa

MAKES about 2 cups   HANDS-ON TIME: 20 minutes   TOTAL TIME: 20 minutes

A vibrant fruit salsa is the perfect partner for simple grilled meat, fish, or chicken. It also works as a dip—take it to a summer cookout and watch it disappear. Add more lime juice, jalapeño, cilantro, and salt and pepper to your taste. When mangoes are out of season, use 1½ cups of diced pineapple or nectarines instead.

1 large mango, peeled, pitted, and diced

½ cup minced red onion

½ cup diced red bell pepper

2 tablespoons finely chopped cilantro

2 tablespoons fresh lime juice

1 tablespoon minced fresh jalapeño

1 teaspoon extra-virgin olive oil

Salt and freshly ground black pepper

In a serving bowl, combine the mango, onion, bell pepper, cilantro, lime juice, jalapeño, oil, and salt and pepper to taste. Serve at room temperature.

NUTRITION AT A GLANCE
Per tablespoon: 8 calories, 0 g fat, 0 g saturated fat, 0 g protein, 2 g carbohydrate, 0 g fiber, 0 mg sodium

TIP: To ripen a mango, leave it at room temperature in a paper bag with an apple until it's fragrant and gently yields when squeezed.

15 MINUTE RECIPE

Chinese Peanut Sauce

MAKES about ¾ cup (2 tablespoons per serving)   HANDS-ON TIME: 5 minutes
TOTAL TIME: 5 minutes

This all-purpose sauce is terrific drizzled over julienned veggies or tossed with whole-wheat noodles. Or try it with Crispy Chicken Fingers, page 144. If you like your sauce spicy, stir in a teaspoon of hot pepper sauce.

- ¼ cup natural no-sugar-added creamy peanut butter
- ¼ cup reduced-sodium soy sauce
- 2 tablespoons minced peeled fresh ginger
- 2 tablespoons rice vinegar

- 2 garlic cloves, minced
- 1 tablespoon dark sesame oil
- 2 teaspoons granular sugar substitute

In a blender or food processor, combine the peanut butter, soy sauce, ginger, vinegar, garlic, sesame oil, and sugar substitute. Process for 1 minute, or until the sauce is the consistency of heavy cream. If too thick, add a little hot water and process again.

NUTRITION AT A GLANCE
Per tablespoon: 49 calories, 4 g fat, 0.5 g saturated fat, 2 g protein, 2 g carbohydrate, 0.5 g fiber, 192 mg sodium

TIP: Make the peanut sauce in advance if you like. It will keep for up to a week in a sealed container in the refrigerator.

Cucumber-Mint Raita

MAKES 1⅓ cups   HANDS-ON TIME: 10 minutes   TOTAL TIME: 10 minutes

**15
MINUTE
RECIPE**

Cooling raita is typically served as an accompaniment to spicy Indian dishes to help put out some of the fire. But it's an equally delicious dip for raw or grilled veggies, or whole-wheat pita on Phase 2. The recipe is easily doubled or tripled and can be refrigerated for a few hours or overnight.

3   medium kirby cucumbers, peeled, halved lengthwise, seeded, and grated

1   cup nonfat plain yogurt

2   tablespoons chopped fresh mint leaves

½   teaspoon ground cumin

Salt and freshly ground black pepper

Wrap the grated cucumber in a kitchen towel and squeeze dry.

In a medium bowl, combine the yogurt, mint, and cumin. Add the cucumber and toss to combine. Season with salt and pepper to taste.

NUTRITION AT A GLANCE

Per tablespoon: 9 calories, 0 g fat, 0 g saturated fat, 1 g protein, 2 g carbohydrate, 0 g fiber, 7 mg sodium

TIP: Use a box grater to grate the cucumber. Squeezing the water from the grated cucumber is an important step; otherwise the raita becomes watery as it sits.

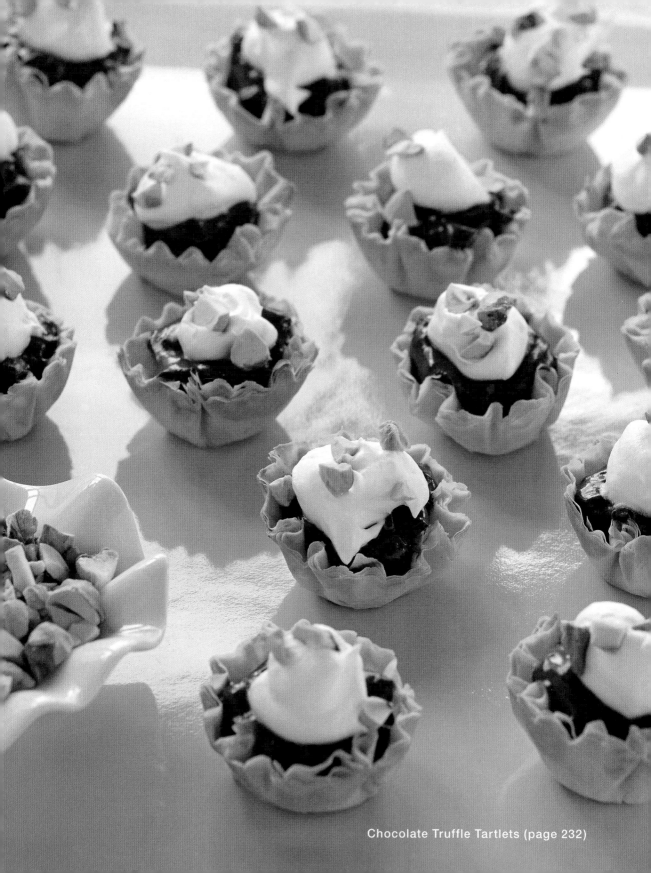

Chocolate Truffle Tartlets (page 232)

DESSERTS

We love dessert, in moderation, on every phase of the South Beach Diet. And there's no reason that you can't prepare a healthy confection in minutes, as this chapter shows. Chocolate lovers will lean toward our dark chocolate bark with walnuts and chocolate truffle tartlets. Fruit lovers will favor grilled summer fruits, mini apple tarts, and bananas with lime cream. And Phase 1 dieters can enjoy macaroons, tofu pudding, and delicious brownies enriched with—of all things—black beans.

The secret to our healthy desserts is a few key substitutions: whole-wheat pastry flour or white whole-wheat flour stands in for regular white flour, and you'll need sugar substitute instead of sugar. And of course, dark bittersweet chocolate is essential!

For more on baking staples, see page 7, and for more great taste-tempting desserts, see the Make-Ahead chapter, page 249.

Chocolate Truffle Tartlets

MAKES 12 tartlets (3 per serving)   **HANDS-ON TIME:** 10 minutes   **TOTAL TIME:** 25 minutes

Look for prebaked mini phyllo shells in the freezer section of your super-market. Because they are so small and low in carbohydrates, we allow them on Phase 2. The shells thaw almost instantly, so there's no need to heat. If you like, add a whole almond, a sprinkling of chopped pistachios, or a sliver of orange as a final garnish. You can refrigerate the tartlets for a few hours or overnight if you want to make them ahead of time.

⅓ cup fat-free half-and-half

1 tablespoon trans-fat-free margarine (vegetable oil spread)

4 tablespoons granular sugar substitute

1 large egg yolk

Pinch salt

2 ounces (2 squares) unsweetened dark baking chocolate, chopped

12 frozen mini phyllo shells, thawed

2 tablespoons no-sugar-added lite whipped topping

In a small saucepan, combine the half-and-half, margarine, and 2 tablespoons of the sugar substitute. Cook over low heat until the mixture is hot and the margarine is melted, about 1 minute.

Meanwhile, in a small bowl, whisk together the remaining 2 tablespoons sugar substitute, the egg yolk, and salt.

Whisk the hot half-and-half mixture into the egg mixture, then whisk back into the saucepan and cook, whisking constantly, for 10 seconds. Remove the pan from the heat, add the chocolate, and cover. Let stand for 5 minutes for the chocolate to melt.

Stir the chocolate mixture to recombine. Spoon 2 teaspoons of the chocolate mixture into each tartlet shell and refrigerate for 10 minutes. To serve, top each with ½ teaspoon whipped topping.

NUTRITION AT A GLANCE
Per tartlet: 64 calories, 5 g fat, 2 g saturated fat, 2 g protein, 5 g carbohydrate, 1 g fiber, 32 mg sodium

Cannoli Pudding

MAKES 4 servings   **HANDS-ON TIME:** 10 minutes   **TOTAL TIME:** 10 minutes

15
MINUTE
RECIPE

Be sure to buy semisweet mini chocolate chips, not milk chocolate, for this dessert modeled after the filling in traditional Italian cannolis. If you're making the dessert for company, garnish each serving with a few extra chocolate chips and a sprinkling of chopped pistachios.

1 container (15 ounces) part-skim ricotta cheese

3 tablespoons granular sugar substitute

2 teaspoons grated orange zest

1 teaspoon vanilla extract

¼ cup mini semisweet chocolate chips

¼ cup coarsely chopped pistachios (1 ounce)

With an electric mixer, beat the ricotta, sugar substitute, orange zest, and vanilla until light and smooth. Fold in the chocolate chips and pistachios.

Spoon the pudding evenly into 4 dessert bowls and serve, or cover and chill to serve later.

NUTRITION AT A GLANCE

Per serving: 247 calories, 15 g fat, 8 g saturated fat, 14 g protein, 16 g carbohydrate, 1 g fiber, 135 mg sodium

Variation: For Phase 1, omit the chocolate chips and add 2 tablespoons unsweetened cocoa powder and 1 additional tablespoon sugar substitute to the ricotta mixture.

Per serving (without chocolate chips): 203 calories, 12 g fat, 6 g saturated fat, 14 g protein, 11 g carbohydrate, 2 g fiber, 134 mg sodium

Glazed Bananas with Lime Cream

MAKES 4 servings   **HANDS-ON TIME: 10 minutes**   **TOTAL TIME: 10 minutes**

Greek yogurt adds richness to this delicious banana dessert, which tastes like a cross between banana cream pie and key lime pie, without the crust!

2 teaspoons grated lime zest

¼ cup fresh lime juice

3 tablespoons plus 2 teaspoons granular sugar substitute

1 tablespoon trans-fat-free margarine (vegetable oil spread)

2 medium bananas, peeled and sliced ½ inch thick

6 ounces nonfat (0%) plain Greek yogurt

Lime twists, for garnish (optional)

In a large skillet, combine 1½ teaspoons of the lime zest, the lime juice, 3 tablespoons of the granular sugar substitute, and the margarine. Cook over low heat until the margarine melts. Add the bananas and cook, turning occasionally, until tender, about 4 minutes.

Meanwhile, in a medium bowl, stir together the remaining ½ teaspoon lime zest and remaining 2 teaspoons sugar substitute. Add the yogurt and stir to blend.

Divide the warm bananas and pan juices evenly among 4 dessert bowls. Spoon the yogurt alongside each serving and garnish with lime twists, if you like.

NUTRITION AT A GLANCE
Per serving: 106 calories, 3 g fat, 1 g saturated fat, 4 g protein, 18 g carbohydrate, 2 g fiber, 39 mg sodium

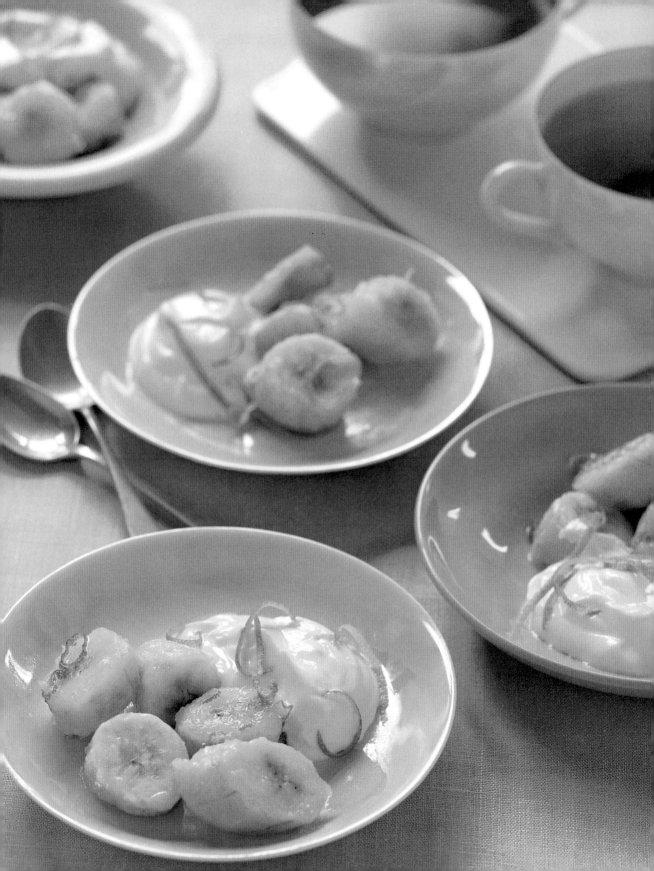

Coconut-Almond Macaroons

MAKES 24 macaroons (3 per serving)   HANDS-ON TIME: 10 minutes   TOTAL TIME: 30 minutes

Almonds add vitamin E, riboflavin, and magnesium to these delicious flourless cookies. For additional filling protein, enjoy the macaroons with a glass of fat-free or 1% milk. On Phase 2, drizzle them with a little melted dark chocolate!

3   ounces slivered almonds
     (generous ⅔ cup)

1¼ cups shredded unsweetened
     coconut

½   cup granular sugar substitute

Generous pinch salt

¼   cup nonfat (0%) plain Greek yogurt

1   large egg white

1   teaspoon vanilla extract

Heat the oven to 325°F. Line a baking sheet with parchment paper or a nonstick liner.

In a mini food processor, pulse the almonds just until ground. Transfer to a medium bowl and add the coconut, sugar substitute, and salt, stirring to combine. Stir in the yogurt, egg white, and vanilla.

Pinch off pieces of dough the size of small walnuts and form into rough balls. Place the balls 2 inches apart on the baking sheet. Bake for 20 minutes, or until golden brown and set. Let cool on the baking sheet.

NUTRITION AT A GLANCE
Per macaroon: 50 calories, 4 g fat, 2 g saturated fat, 1 g protein, 2 g carbohydrate, 1 g fiber, 17 mg sodium

Silken Chocolate Pudding

MAKES 4 (½-cup) servings HANDS-ON TIME: 10 minutes TOTAL TIME: 10 minutes

15 MINUTE RECIPE

Silken tofu has a softer consistency than regular tofu and is perfect for this creamy Phase 1 pudding. It comes in soft, medium, firm, and extra-firm consistencies; be sure to buy the soft type to use here.

1 package (16 ounces) soft silken tofu, drained

2 tablespoons unsweetened cocoa powder

¼ cup granular sugar substitute

1 teaspoon vanilla extract

¼ teaspoon salt

4 tablespoons no-sugar-added lite whipped topping

2 tablespoons dry-roasted raw peanuts, chopped

In a food processor or blender, combine the tofu, cocoa powder, sugar substitute, vanilla, and salt. Purée until smooth.

Spoon the pudding into 4 dessert dishes, dollop each serving with 1 tablespoon whipped topping, and sprinkle each evenly with chopped peanuts. Serve right away or chill to serve later (but don't add the topping and peanuts until ready to serve).

NUTRITION AT A GLANCE

Per serving: 124 calories, 6 g fat, 1 g saturated fat, 7 g protein, 10 g carbohydrate, 1 g fiber, 152 mg sodium

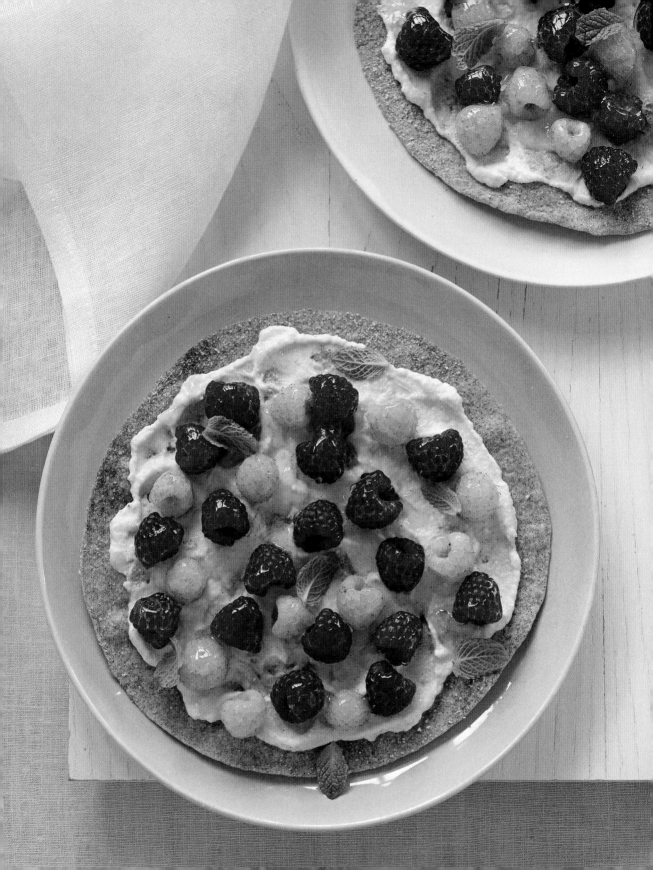

Apricot-Berry Dessert Pizza

MAKES 4 pizzas   **HANDS-ON TIME: 10 minutes**   **TOTAL TIME: 15 minutes**

Easy and elegant, these dessert pizzas are a novel way to use tortillas. The
addition of cardamom, along with lemon zest and apricot jam, gives the pizzas
a Mediterranean flavor. Use any of your favorite berries for the topping.

4 (8-inch) whole-wheat flour tortillas

4 teaspoons trans-fat-free margarine
(vegetable oil spread), melted

4 teaspoons granular sugar
substitute

½ teaspoon ground cinnamon

1⅓ cups part-skim ricotta cheese

9 teaspoons sugar-free apricot jam

1 teaspoon grated lemon zest

½ teaspoon ground cardamom

4 cups yellow and red raspberries,
or blueberries, or a mixture

Fresh mint leaves, for garnish
(optional)

Heat the oven to 400°F. Place the tortillas on 2 baking sheets. Brush with the
melted margarine and sprinkle evenly with the sugar substitute and
cinnamon. Bake for 7 to 10 minutes, until crisp. Cool briefly.

Meanwhile, in a medium bowl, stir together the ricotta, 4 teaspoons of
the apricot jam, the lemon zest, and cardamom.

Divide the ricotta mixture among the 4 tortillas, spreading it almost to
the edges.

In a small saucepan, heat the remaining 5 teaspoons jam over low heat
until melted. Scatter the berries over the pizzas and brush the berries with the
melted jam. Garnish with mint leaves, if using. Serve warm.

NUTRITION AT A GLANCE
Per pizza: 346 calories, 13 g fat, 5 g saturated fat, 14 g protein, 45 g carbohydrate, 12 g fiber,
434 mg sodium

Mini Apple Tarts

MAKES 15 mini tarts (3 per serving)   HANDS-ON TIME: 15 minutes   TOTAL TIME: 20 minutes

There's no need to heat the prebaked tart shells for this recipe. However, if you prefer serving warm tarts, spoon the apple mixture into the shells while it is still warm, then top with the cream cheese mixture. Be sure to choose sweet, not tart, apples. For more information on agave nectar, see page 99.

1 tablespoon trans-fat-free margarine (vegetable oil spread)

2 medium red apples, peeled, quartered, cored, and thinly sliced

3 ounces reduced-fat cream cheese

1 tablespoon light agave nectar or 2 teaspoons granular sugar substitute

15 frozen mini phyllo shells, thawed

In a large nonstick skillet, melt the margarine over medium heat. Add the apples and cook, tossing frequently, until softened and golden brown, 5 to 7 minutes. Transfer to a plate and cool for 5 minutes.

Meanwhile, in a small bowl, stir together the cream cheese and agave nectar.

Spoon the cream cheese mixture evenly into the tart shells. Top with the apples and serve.

NUTRITION AT A GLANCE
Per tart: 53 calories, 2.5 g fat, 1 g saturated fat, 1 g protein, 7 g carbohydrate, 2 g fiber, 41 mg sodium

Strawberry Fool

MAKES 4 servings   HANDS-ON TIME: 5 minutes   TOTAL TIME: 30 minutes

If you purée the frozen strawberries just before you sit down to dinner, they will thaw while you eat. Then, after dinner, it takes only about 5 minutes to whip together this delicious dessert.

- 1 cup frozen unsweetened strawberries (5 ounces)
- 4 teaspoons granular sugar substitute
- 1½ cups nonfat (0%) plain Greek yogurt
- ½ teaspoon vanilla extract
- ½ cup no-sugar-added lite whipped topping

In a food processor, pulse the strawberries on and off to break them up, then process until smooth. Add 2 teaspoons of the sugar substitute and pulse to combine. Let sit in the food processor for 20 to 25 minutes to thaw completely.

Meanwhile, in a medium bowl, whisk the Greek yogurt to lighten, then whisk in the vanilla and remaining 2 teaspoons sugar substitute. Whisk in the whipped topping.

Process the strawberry purée again to loosen, then pour over the yogurt mixture. Gently fold in with a rubber spatula, leaving streaks of strawberry.

Divide the fool evenly among 4 dessert dishes and serve.

NUTRITION AT A GLANCE
Per serving: 101 calories, 0 g fat, 0 g saturated fat, 7 g protein, 13 g carbohydrate, 1 g fiber, 32 mg sodium

Dark Chocolate Bark with Walnuts

MAKES 20 pieces (2 per serving)   HANDS-ON TIME: 10 minutes   TOTAL TIME: 30 minutes

On Phase 2 of the South Beach Diet you can occasionally enjoy a small amount of antioxidant-rich dark chocolate. This dessert (which also features heart-healthy walnuts) will certainly satisfy any chocolate lover's dreams.

¾ cup coarsely chopped walnuts

6 ounces bittersweet dark chocolate, finely chopped

Heat the oven to 350°F. Place the walnuts on a baking sheet and toast for 8 minutes, or until fragrant. Cool, then coarsely chop.

Place 4 ounces of the chopped chocolate in a medium glass bowl. Microwave on high for 30 seconds. Stir, then microwave for 30 seconds longer, or until just melted. (If the chocolate hasn't melted, microwave an additional 20 seconds.) Add the remaining chocolate to the bowl, stirring until melted. Stir in the walnuts.

Line a baking sheet with parchment paper or waxed paper. Spread the warm chocolate mixture onto the sheet into a 6 × 9-inch rectangle. Refrigerate for 10 minutes, or until firm but not brittle. Cut or break into about 20 jagged pieces and serve, or refrigerate for later (the bark will keep for 2 weeks in an airtight container).

NUTRITION AT A GLANCE
Per piece: 71 calories, 6.5 g fat, 2 g saturated fat, 1 g protein, 5 g carbohydrate, 1 g fiber, 0 mg sodium

TIP: If you don't have a microwave oven, melt the chocolate in the top of a double boiler over simmering water.

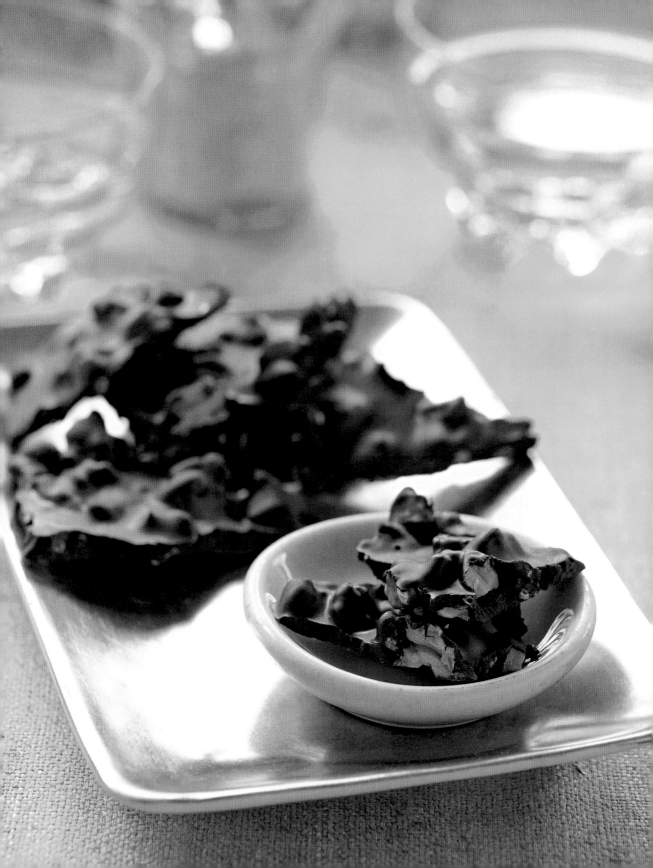

15 MINUTE RECIPE

Grilled Summer Fruits

MAKES 4 servings   **HANDS-ON TIME: 10 minutes**   **TOTAL TIME: 15 minutes**

Grilling fruit caramelizes its natural sugars, enhancing the flavor. Be sure to monitor the grilling carefully so the skin doesn't burn and the fruit doesn't become mushy. Besides plums and nectarines, other fruits that lend themselves to grilling include bananas, peaches, mangoes, apples, and pears. (Harder fruits such as apples and pears will take longer to grill than softer fruits.)

2 teaspoons extra-virgin olive oil, plus oil for grill rack

1 teaspoon fresh lemon juice

   Pinch ground cinnamon, allspice, or nutmeg (optional)

2 ripe plums, halved and pitted

2 ripe nectarines, halved and pitted

4 tablespoons no-sugar-added lite whipped topping (optional)

Heat a grill to medium.

In a cup, combine the oil, lemon juice, and spice (if using). Brush over the cut sides of the plums and nectarines.

Lightly coat the grill rack with oil. Place the plums and nectarines, cut side down, on the rack. Grill, uncovered, turning once, until the fruit is tender and lightly browned, about 5 minutes depending on the ripeness of the fruit. Top each fruit half with ½ tablespoon whipped topping, if using.

NUTRITION AT A GLANCE
Per serving: 68 calories, 3 g fat, 0.4 g saturated fat, 1 g protein, 11 g carbohydrate, 2 g fiber, 0 mg sodium

TIP: Make sure you clean the grill well so the fruit doesn't take on the flavor of burgers or other meats, or use a clean grill topper.

Black Bean Brownies

MAKES 36 brownies (3 per serving) HANDS-ON TIME: 5 minutes TOTAL TIME: 30 minutes

This healthy twist on a classic brownie recipe was suggested by a devoted South Beach dieter. It substitutes fiber-rich black beans and heart-healthy olive oil for the usual butter. When Dr. Agatston (a known chocolate lover) sampled the brownies, he was surprised by how moist and delicious they were and was delighted to learn that beans were the "secret ingredient." You can serve the brownies hot from the pan or at room temperature.

1 can (15.5 ounces) black beans, drained and rinsed

4 large eggs

2 tablespoons extra-virgin olive oil

1 teaspoon vanilla extract

1 cup granular sugar substitute

3 tablespoons unsweetened cocoa powder, preferably dark

1 teaspoon baking powder

¼ teaspoon salt

36 small pecan halves or walnut pieces (about 1.5 ounces)

Heat the oven to 350°F. Lightly coat an 8 × 8-inch baking pan with cooking spray.

In a blender or food processor, combine the beans, eggs, oil, vanilla, sugar substitute, cocoa powder, baking powder, and salt. Process until smooth.

Scrape the batter into the pan and arrange the nuts in even rows, 6 across and 6 down. Bake for 25 to 30 minutes, until a toothpick inserted in the center comes out clean. Cut into 36 squares with a nut piece in the center of each.

NUTRITION AT A GLANCE
Per brownie: 34 calories, 2 g fat, 0.4 g saturated fat, 1 g protein, 2 g carbohydrate, 1 g fiber, 66 mg sodium

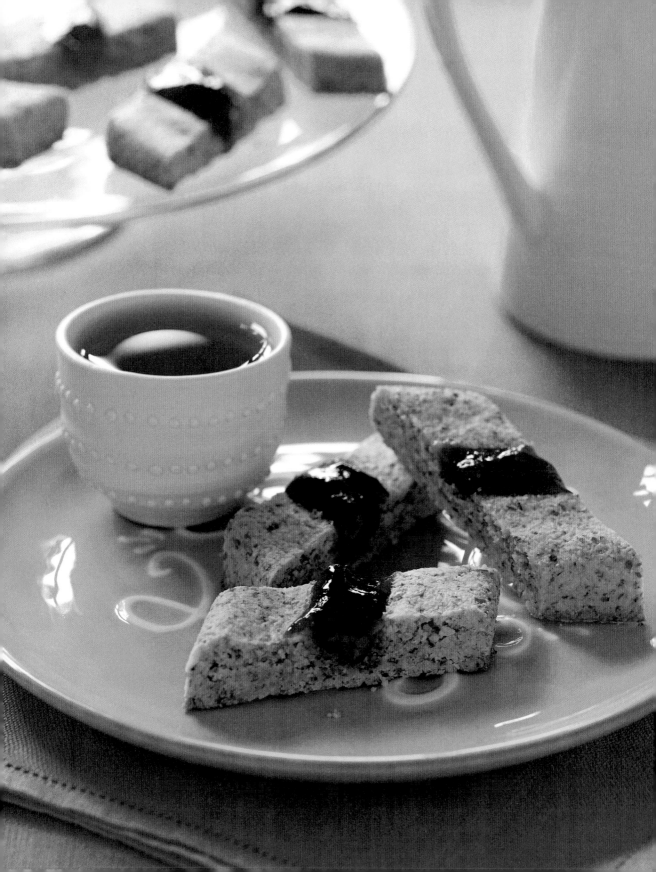

Almond-Jam Bars

MAKES 27 bars (3 per serving) **HANDS-ON TIME: 10 minutes** **TOTAL TIME: 30 minutes**

These delicious Phase 1 dessert bars are a healthy variation on the popular jam-filled thumbprint cookies. Here ground almonds take the place of flour. Use whatever flavor of sugar-free jam you like best (it's considered a Sweet Treat on Phase 1).

1 cup natural unblanched almonds (5 ounces)

¼ cup granular sugar substitute

¼ teaspoon salt

1 large egg white

¼ cup sugar-free jam

Heat the oven to 375°F. Line a large baking sheet with parchment.

In a food processor, process the almonds, sugar substitute, and salt until finely ground. Add the egg white and process until the mixture forms a paste.

Transfer the dough to the baking sheet and shape into a 14 × 2-inch log. With a moistened thumb, make a ¼-inch-deep trench down the length of the log. Bake for 12 to 15 minutes, until lightly golden and set.

A few minutes before the log comes out of the oven, in a small saucepan, heat the jam over low heat until melted.

Once the log is baked, immediately spoon the jam along the trench. Cool the log on the baking sheet for 10 minutes before cutting crosswise on an angle into 27 bars, each a scant ½ inch thick.

NUTRITION AT A GLANCE
Per bar: 34 calories, 3 g fat, 0 g saturated fat, 1 g protein, 2 g carbohydrate, 1 g fiber, 24 mg sodium

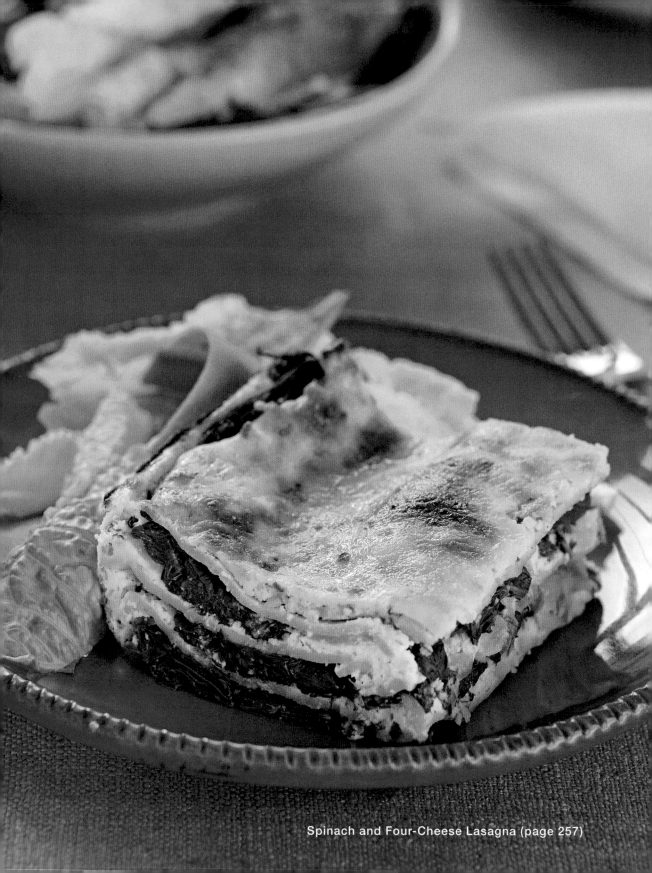

Spinach and Four-Cheese Lasagna (page 257)

MAKE-AHEAD DISHES

Sometimes the easiest dishes for busy days are those you can start well in advance, so they are ready when you are. The breakfasts, breads, soups, stews, casseroles, and desserts in this chapter may take a bit (or a lot) longer than 30 minutes to prepare, thanks to the time needed for chilling, marinating, or slow cooking. But virtually all of the additional time is unattended, and in return you often get more than one meal for your efforts, as well as a great dining experience.

The spinach and cheese lasagna, beef stew, chicken chili, salmon burgers, and toaster waffles, for example, all freeze well for meals down the road (spend a Saturday getting ahead on a few of them). The black bean soup simmers all day in a slow cooker and is ready when you get home. The steel-cut oatmeal slow cooks all night for a quick, hearty, and healthy morning meal. And the cheesecake, panna cotta, and sherbet just need time to set. Whether you're cooking weekday meals for your family or making a special dinner for special friends, these premade dishes will come in handy time and again.

Overnight Oatmeal

MAKES 8 (1-cup) servings   HANDS-ON TIME: 15 minutes   TOTAL TIME: 6 to 8 hours

You'll need a 2-quart slow cooker for this recipe. If you have a bigger cooker, you can use a 2-quart baking dish set into it. This oatmeal makes enough for eight and it keeps for up to a week, which makes it a great make-ahead, grab-and-go breakfast. Pack the oatmeal into microwavable containers that will hold a 1-cup serving plus a little room for milk. Then at breakfast time, just add a little fat-free or 1% milk and reheat for 45 seconds to 1 minute in a microwave oven.

1 tablespoon trans-fat-free margarine (vegetable oil spread)

1 cup steel-cut oats

1 cup chopped dried apples (3 ounces)

3 tablespoons granular sugar substitute

1 teaspoon ground cinnamon

¼ teaspoon salt

½ cup fat-free or 1% milk

½ teaspoon vanilla extract

Using the margarine, grease the bottom and 2 inches up the sides of the liner of a 2-quart electric slow cooker or grease a 2-quart baking dish that will fit into the slow cooker. If using a baking dish, add ½ inch of water to the liner of the cooker.

Add the oats, apples, sugar substitute, cinnamon, and salt to the liner or baking dish. Gently add 3½ cups water, the milk, and vanilla, but do not stir. Cover and cook on low heat for 6 to 8 hours.

NUTRITION AT A GLANCE
Per serving: 128 calories, 3 g fat, 0.4 g saturated fat, 4 g protein, 22 g carbohydrate, 5 g fiber, 162 mg sodium

Multigrain Toaster Waffles

MAKES 12 (4-inch) waffles (2 per serving)   HANDS-ON TIME: 25 minutes   TOTAL TIME: 25 minutes

Premade multigrain waffles go straight from the freezer to the toaster for a fast and healthy start to a rush, rush day. Spread two with some nut butter and pack for a grab-and-go breakfast. You can also make this recipe as a dry mix, so you'll quickly be able to whip up a batch of waffles whenever you want. Double or triple the recipe and keep the mix in the refrigerator indefinitely. Look for buttermilk powder with the baking ingredients in your supermarket. For information on flaxmeal, see page 147.

1½ cups whole-wheat flour

¼ cup flaxmeal

¼ cup quick-cooking oats

⅓ cup buttermilk powder or instant nonfat dry milk

1 tablespoon baking powder

2 teaspoons granular sugar substitute

½ teaspoon ground cinnamon (optional)

½ teaspoon salt

2 large eggs

1½ tablespoons canola oil or extra-virgin olive oil

Heat a waffle iron, preferably nonstick.

In a medium bowl, stir together the flour, flaxmeal, oats, buttermilk powder, baking powder, sugar substitute, cinnamon (if using), and salt.

Make a well in the middle of the flour mixture. Add the eggs and lightly beat with a fork. Add 1½ cups water and the oil and blend, pulling the batter in from the sides of the bowl as you mix.

Ladle some batter into the center of the waffle iron until it spreads to 1 inch from the edges. (The amount will vary with the size of the waffle iron. If you're using a 4-square waffle iron, it will be about 1 cup batter per batch.) Cover and cook according to the waffle maker's instructions. Continue until all the batter is used up. As they are cooked, transfer the waffles to a wire rack and let cool to room temperature.

Cut each waffle into 4 pieces, place on a baking sheet, and freeze until solid. Store in resealable plastic freezer bags for up to 6 months. Reheat straight from the freezer in a toaster or toaster oven.

NUTRITION AT A GLANCE
Per waffle: 103 calories, 4 g fat, 0.4 g saturated fat, 4 g protein, 14 g carbohydrate, 2 g fiber, 227 mg sodium

Whole-Wheat Avocado Bread

MAKES 10 servings (1 piece per serving)   HANDS-ON TIME: 10 minutes   TOTAL TIME: 55 minutes

Help yourself to this moist, rich, and slightly sweet tea bread instead of a sugary high-fat muffin. It's got whole-grain goodness and healthy monounsaturated fat from the avocados in every delicious bite. Make the bread when you have some free time, wrap it well, and enjoy it for up to a week.

2   cups whole-wheat pastry flour

¾   cup granular sugar substitute

¾   teaspoon baking soda

½   teaspoon salt

2   ripe avocados, pitted, peeled, and mashed

½   cup nonfat plain yogurt or light (1.5%) buttermilk

2   large eggs

2   tablespoons canola oil

1   teaspoon vanilla extract

Heat the oven to 350°F. Lightly coat the bottom of a 9 × 5-inch loaf pan with cooking spray.

In a large bowl, combine the flour, sugar substitute, baking soda, and salt.

In a medium bowl, stir together the avocados, yogurt, eggs, oil, and vanilla. Lightly fold the mixture into the dry ingredients until just combined. The batter will be thick and chunky.

Scrape the batter into the pan and spread evenly. Bake for 40 minutes, or until golden on top and a toothpick inserted in the center comes out clean. Cool in the pan for 5 minutes, then transfer to a wire rack. Store leftover bread, tightly wrapped, at room temperature.

NUTRITION AT A GLANCE
Per serving: 185 calories, 8 g fat, 1 g saturated fat, 5 g protein, 23 g carbohydrate, 4 g fiber, 234 mg sodium

TIP: Unlike bananas used for quick bread, you want the avocados to be ripe but not black for this recipe.

Italian-Style Black Bean Soup

MAKES 8 servings   HANDS-ON TIME: 25 minutes   TOTAL TIME: 8 hours, plus bean soaking time

You'll need a 5- to 6-quart slow cooker for this full-bodied soup. Serve it with your choice of garnishes and a simple salad of mixed greens for a satisfying lunch or dinner. On Phase 2, enjoy it with some whole-grain Italian bread.

1   pound dried black beans

1   tablespoon extra-virgin olive oil

2   medium red bell peppers, finely chopped

1   large onion, finely chopped

3   celery stalks, finely chopped

5   garlic cloves, minced

1½ tablespoons ground cumin

¼   teaspoon red pepper flakes

Salt and freshly ground black pepper

6   cups lower-sodium vegetable broth

2   bay leaves

⅛   teaspoon baking soda

2   tablespoons fresh lime juice

Lime wedges, chopped fresh cilantro, diced red onion, diced avocado, and/or reduced-fat sour cream, for garnish

Place the beans in a large bowl. Cover with water and soak for at least 6 hours or overnight. Drain.

In a large saucepan, heat the oil over medium-high heat. Add the bell peppers, onion, and celery and cook until softened, about 10 minutes.

Add the garlic, cumin, red pepper flakes, and salt and black pepper to taste. Cook over medium-low heat, stirring constantly, until fragrant, about 2 minutes. Stir in the broth and remove from the heat.

In a 5- to 6-quart slow cooker, combine the beans, bay leaves, baking soda, and a pinch of salt. Pour the vegetable mixture over the beans. Cover and cook over high heat for about 5 hours, or until the beans are creamy. (Or cook for 8 hours on low heat.)

Discard the bay leaves. Ladle about 1½ cups of the soup into a food processor or blender (or use an immersion blender and a large bowl) and process until smooth. Return to the slow cooker and stir in the lime juice. Serve hot with your favorite garnishes.

NUTRITION AT A GLANCE
Per serving: 248 calories, 2 g fat, 0.3 g saturated fat, 12 g protein, 42 g carbohydrate, 7 g fiber, 141 mg sodium

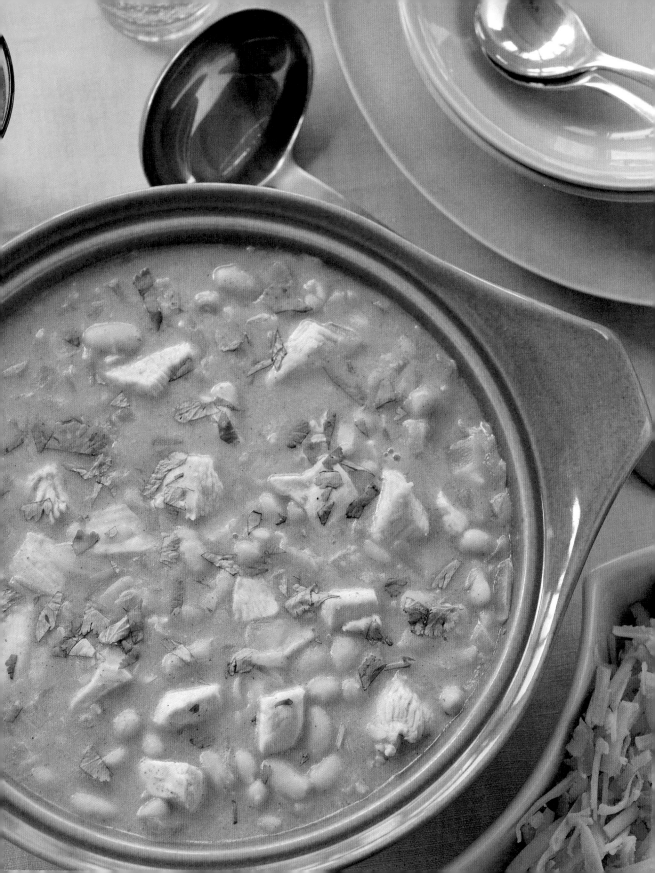

White Chipotle Chicken Chili

MAKES 8 (1½-cup) servings   **HANDS-ON TIME: 30 minutes**   **TOTAL TIME: 35 minutes**

This is a great dish to make-ahead when you know company is coming (it freezes really well). Here it serves eight, but it can easily be doubled for a bigger crowd. To freeze the chili for individual meals, let it come to room temperature, then ladle into 2-cup freezer containers. To serve, thaw the chili and reheat over low heat or in the microwave.

2 tablespoons extra-virgin olive oil	Salt
3 medium onions, chopped	3 cans (19 ounces each) cannellini beans, drained and rinsed
4 large garlic cloves, minced	
2½ pounds boneless, skinless chicken breasts, cut into 1-inch chunks	3 cups lower-sodium chicken broth
	½ cup fat-free half-and-half
1 tablespoon chipotle chile powder or chili seasoning	½ cup reduced-fat shredded Cheddar cheese (2 ounces)
4 teaspoons ground cumin	¼ cup chopped fresh cilantro

In a large Dutch oven, heat the oil over medium-low heat. Add the onions and cook, stirring occasionally, until beginning to soften, 4 to 5 minutes.

Push the onions to one side of the pan, add the chicken, and sprinkle with the chipotle chile powder, cumin, and salt to taste. Cook, stirring, until most of the chicken is opaque on the outside, 5 to 6 minutes.

Stir in 3 cups of the beans and 2 cups of the broth. Increase the heat to medium-high and bring to a simmer. Partially cover and cook until the chicken is cooked through, about 8 minutes.

Meanwhile, in a food processor, combine the remaining beans and remaining 1 cup broth. Process to a smooth purée.

Stir the bean purée and half-and-half into the soup. Divide the soup among 4 bowls and serve hot sprinkled with cheese and cilantro.

NUTRITION AT A GLANCE
Per serving: 371 calories, 9 g fat, 3 g saturated fat, 43 g protein, 27 g carbohydrate, 7 g fiber, 483 mg sodium

TIP: If you want to prepare your own cooked white beans for this recipe, you'll need 4½ cups (from 2¼ cups dried).

Vegetable Tart

MAKES 8 servings   HANDS-ON TIME: 35 minutes   TOTAL TIME: 1 hour 50 minutes

The tart shells call for white whole-wheat flour, available in supermarkets. Lighter and milder than traditional whole-wheat flour, it still has just as much fiber.

TART SHELL

- 1½ cups white whole-wheat flour
- 2 tablespoons chopped fresh chives, parsley, and/or thyme
- 1 teaspoon salt
- ¼ cup extra-virgin olive oil
- 10 tablespoons ice water

FILLING

- 2 teaspoons extra-virgin olive oil
- 2 large shallots, chopped
- 1½ cups thinly sliced shiitake mushroom caps
- ½ pound medium asparagus, cut into 1-inch pieces
- 1 package (10 ounces) frozen spinach, thawed and squeezed of excess liquid
- ½ cup part-skim ricotta cheese
- 3 large eggs
- Salt and freshly ground black pepper
- ½ cup shredded reduced-fat Swiss cheese (2 ounces)

Heat the oven to 325°F. Coat a 9-inch tart pan with cooking spray.

For the tart shell: In a large bowl, stir together the flour, herbs, and salt. Blend in the oil with your fingers. Add the water, a couple of tablespoons at a time, blending until a ball forms. Knead a few times until smooth. Pat into a disk, wrap in plastic, and refrigerate for 15 minutes.

Meanwhile, to make the filling: In a large nonstick skillet, heat the oil over medium-high heat. Add the shallots and cook for 2 minutes. Add the mushrooms and cook for 3 minutes. Add the asparagus and cook for 3 minutes. Stir in the spinach.

Roll the dough out to a 12-inch circle. Press into the tart pan, tucking the edges under. Prick the dough with a fork several times. Bake for 10 minutes, or until the crust looks dry. Let cool briefly. Increase the oven temperature to 350°F.

In a large bowl, stir together the ricotta, eggs, vegetable mixture, and salt and pepper to taste. Spread in the tart shell. Top with the Swiss cheese. Bake for 50 to 55 minutes, until lightly browned. Serve warm or at room temperature.

NUTRITION AT A GLANCE

Per serving: 256 calories, 13 g fat, 3 g saturated fat, 12 g protein, 6 g carbohydrate, 4 g fiber, 376 mg sodium

Spinach and Four-Cheese Lasagna

MAKES 8 servings   HANDS-ON TIME: 25 minutes   TOTAL TIME: 1 hour 40 minutes

This dish freezes perfectly. Allow it to cool in the pan first.

- 9 whole-wheat lasagna noodles
- 2 packages (16 ounces each) prewashed baby spinach
- 2 teaspoons extra-virgin olive oil
- 3 medium onions, coarsely chopped

  Salt and freshly ground black pepper
- 1 container (15 ounces) part-skim ricotta cheese
- 1 container (8 ounces) 1% whipped cottage cheese

- ½ cup plus 2 tablespoons grated Parmesan cheese
- 4 large eggs
- ¼ cup chopped fresh parsley
- 3 garlic cloves, minced
- 1½ teaspoons dried oregano
- ¼ teaspoon ground nutmeg
- ½ cup shredded part-skim mozzarella cheese

Heat the oven to 350°F. Coat a 9 × 13-inch baking dish with cooking spray. In a large pot of lightly salted boiling water, cook the noodles according to package directions. Using tongs, transfer the noodles to a colander and rinse under cold water.

In the same pot of boiling water, in 2 batches, blanch the spinach for 30 seconds. Using a strainer, remove the spinach and rinse under cold water. Squeeze as much water as possible from the spinach and set aside.

In a large nonstick skillet, heat the oil over medium heat. Add the onions and cook, stirring occasionally, until lightly browned, about 6 minutes.

Off the heat, add the spinach and stir. Season with salt and pepper.

In a large bowl, combine the ricotta, cottage cheese, ½ cup Parmesan, the eggs, parsley, garlic, oregano, and nutmeg. Season with salt and pepper.

Spread 1 cup spinach over the bottom of the pan. Top with 3 noodles and 1½ cups cheese mixture. Top with 2 cups spinach, 3 noodles, 1½ cups cheese mixture, and the remaining spinach, noodles, and cheese mixture. Sprinkle with the mozzarella and remaining 2 tablespoons Parmesan.

Bake for 45 minutes, or until golden. Let sit for 15 minutes before cutting.

NUTRITION AT A GLANCE
Per serving: 359 calories, 13 g fat, 7 g saturated fat, 23 g protein, 39 g carbohydrate, 10 g fiber, 661 mg sodium

Dijon Salmon Burgers

MAKES 4 servings   HANDS-ON TIME: 15 minutes   TOTAL TIME: 1 hour

Make a double batch of these delicious burgers to freeze for future use. Simply wrap the uncooked burgers individually before freezing, then thaw when ready to use and cook as below. On Phase 2, enjoy the burger on a whole-wheat bun.

3   pouches (6 ounces each) boneless, skinless pink salmon

3   scallions, chopped

2   tablespoons chopped fresh dill or tarragon

1   tablespoon nonpareil capers, drained and rinsed (optional)

1   tablespoon fresh lemon juice

1   teaspoon Dijon mustard

¼   teaspoon salt

½   teaspoon freshly ground black pepper

¼   cup reduced-fat mayonnaise

1   large egg

4   teaspoons extra-virgin olive oil

Lettuce leaves, for serving

Sliced tomato, red onion, and cucumber, for toppings (optional)

In a medium bowl, combine the salmon, scallions, dill, capers (if using), lemon juice, mustard, salt, and pepper. Fold in the mayonnaise and egg. Cover and refrigerate for at least 30 minutes.

When ready to cook, form the salmon mixture into 4 (1-inch-thick) patties, pressing the mixture together so the patties are firm.

In a large, heavy skillet, heat the oil over medium-high heat. Add the patties and cook until well browned on both sides and just firm to the touch, about 6 minutes per side.

Serve each burger on a bed of lettuce with tomato, red onion, and cucumber for toppings, if desired.

NUTRITION AT A GLANCE

Per serving: 251 calories, 13 g fat, 2 g saturated fat, 34 g protein, 3 g carbohydrate, 0.4 g fiber, 725 mg sodium

Per serving (with bun): 366 calories, 15 g fat, 2 g saturated fat, 37 g protein, 25 g carbohydrate, 4 g fiber, 930 mg sodium

TIP: The salmon mixture is moist and loose, so be sure to refrigerate it before forming the patties to help them hold together during cooking. The burgers firm up once the first side is cooked.

Grilled Tandoori Chicken

MAKES 4 servings   HANDS-ON TIME: 15 minutes   TOTAL TIME: 1 hour or overnight

In India, this popular yogurt-and-spice-marinated chicken would cook in a superhot tandoor oven. Here, it cooks on the grill or under the broiler. Serve the chicken warm or at room temperature with cooling Cucumber-Mint Raita (page 229) or Mango Salsa (page 227).

4 (5-ounce) boneless, skinless chicken breast halves	1 teaspoon ground cumin
Salt	1 teaspoon garam masala
2 tablespoons fresh lemon juice	1 teaspoon paprika
2 cups nonfat plain yogurt	1 teaspoon turmeric

Place the chicken in a shallow glass bowl or pie plate. Using a sharp knife, cut 3 shallow slashes into each breast. Sprinkle the breasts lightly with salt, then drizzle with the lemon juice.

In a medium bowl, combine the yogurt, cumin, garam masala, paprika, and turmeric. Spoon over the chicken and turn the breasts to coat well. Cover and marinate in the refrigerator for 1 hour, or up to 12 hours.

Heat a grill to medium-high or heat the broiler. Remove the chicken from the dish, but do not wipe off. Grill or broil the chicken about 5 minutes per side, until cooked through but still juicy. (Broiling may take a little longer.) Serve warm or at room temperature.

NUTRITION AT A GLANCE
Per serving: 188 calories, 2 g fat, 0.5 g saturated fat, 35 g protein, 6 g carbohydrate, 0.5 g fiber, 132 mg sodium

TIPS: The longer the chicken marinates, the deeper the flavor. For more on garam masala, see page 102.

Cook Once, Eat Twice

Grill a double batch and the next day toss the extra with watercress, grape tomatoes, some red onion, and a dressing of extra-virgin olive oil and vinegar for a salad.

Beef Burgundy

MAKES 8 servings   HANDS-ON TIME: 30 minutes   TOTAL TIME: 2 hours

When it's chilly outside, what better way to entertain friends than with a heart-warming stew? If you don't want to serve it right away, freeze the stew in plastic containers, then thaw in the refrigerator and reheat on the stovetop or in a microwave oven at a later date.

5 tablespoons extra-virgin olive oil

2 pounds beef top round, well trimmed and cut into ½-inch pieces

4 medium onions, chopped

4 medium carrots, cut crosswise into ½-inch-thick rounds

1 container (10 ounces) white mushrooms, quartered

5 garlic cloves, smashed and peeled

2 whole sprigs fresh rosemary, plus additional cut-up sprigs for garnish

1 cup red wine

1 can (28 ounces) diced tomatoes, with juice

¼ cup tomato paste

Salt and freshly ground black pepper

In a Dutch oven or large saucepan, heat the oil over medium-high heat. Add half the beef and cook until browned on the outside, about 5 minutes. Transfer to a plate and repeat with the remaining beef.

Reduce the heat to medium and add the onions. Cook, scraping up any brown bits, until the onions are softened, about 3 minutes.

Add the carrots, mushrooms, garlic, and rosemary stems. Continue to cook until the mushrooms start giving off their juice, about 3 minutes longer.

Pour the wine over the vegetables, stir well, and bring to a boil. Stir in the tomatoes and their juice, tomato paste, and 2 cups water. Return the beef to the pan and stir to combine.

Cover the pan, leaving the cover slightly ajar, and simmer the stew for 1 hour over medium-low heat. Season with salt and pepper to taste and continue to cook for 30 minutes longer, or until the carrots and meat are tender. Remove the rosemary sprigs and discard. Serve the stew hot.

NUTRITION AT A GLANCE
Per serving: 367 calories, 18 g fat, 5 g saturated fat, 28 g protein, 15 g carbohydrate, 3 g fiber, 388 mg sodium

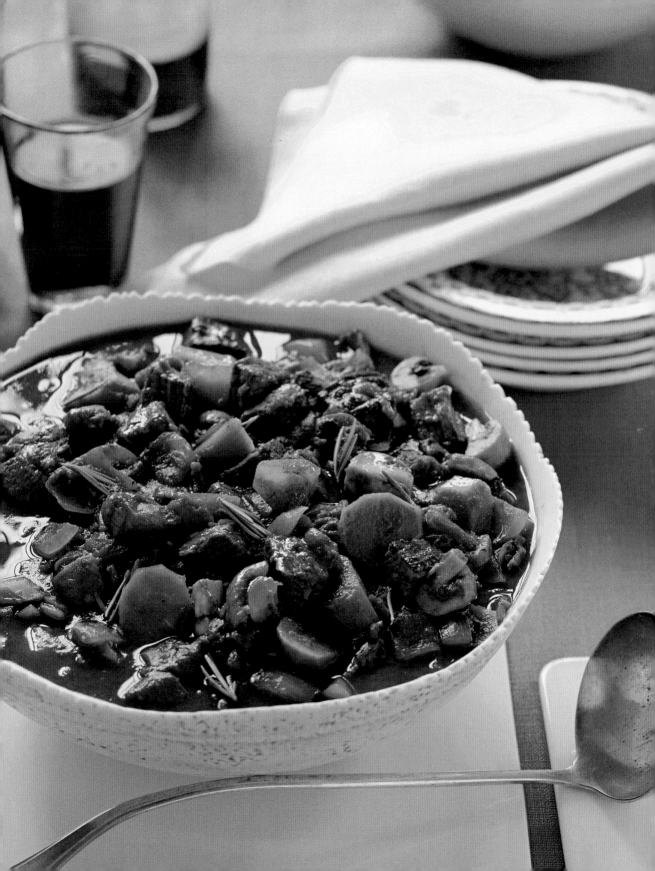

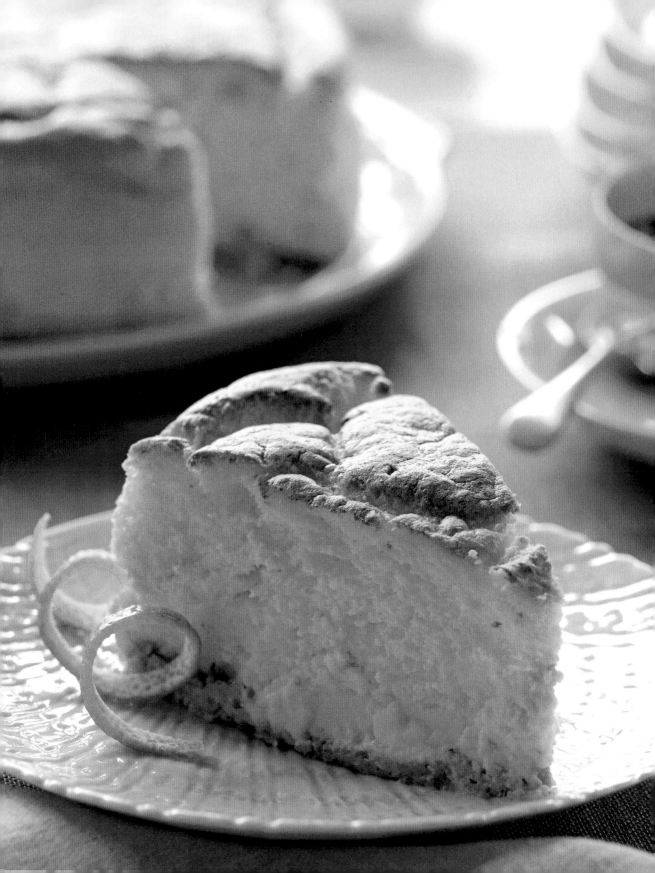

Orange-Almond Ricotta Cheesecake

MAKES 12 servings   HANDS-ON TIME: 15 minutes   TOTAL TIME: 1 hour 20 minutes, plus chill time

This light Italian-style cheesecake is a lovely Phase 2 dessert and an ideal make-ahead for a party. Ground almonds in the crust and almond extract in the batter are a nice flavor contrast to the orange.

- ½ cup slivered almonds
- ⅓ cup graham cracker crumbs
- 6 large eggs, separated
- ¾ teaspoon cream of tartar
- ⅓ cup granular sugar substitute
- 1 tablespoon vanilla extract

- 1 teaspoon almond extract
- 1 container (32 ounces) part-skim ricotta cheese
- 2 teaspoons finely grated orange zest
- ¼ cup fresh orange juice
- Orange twists, for garnish (optional)

Position a rack in the middle of the oven and heat the oven to 275°F. Lightly coat a 9-inch springform pan with cooking spray. Spread the almonds on a baking sheet and toast for 10 to 12 minutes, or until light golden. Let cool.

In a food processor, pulse the cooled almonds until finely ground. Add the cracker crumbs and pulse to combine. Increase the oven temperature to 325°F.

In a large metal bowl, with an electric mixer at high speed, beat the egg whites until frothy, about 1 minute. Add the cream of tartar and continue to beat until stiff peaks form, about 3 minutes longer.

In a separate large bowl, beat the egg yolks, sugar substitute, and vanilla and almond extracts for 1 minute. Add the ricotta, orange zest, and orange juice. Beat on high until smooth. Gently fold one-third of the whites into the yolk mixture, then add the rest of the whites and gently fold until well combined. Spread the crumb mixture over the bottom of the pan. Pour the batter into the pan and place the pan on a baking sheet. Bake for 1 hour and 10 minutes, or until the cake is golden and mostly set. Cool completely.

Run a knife around the edge and release the cake from the pan. Chill, loosely covered, for 4 hours or overnight. Serve chilled, garnished with orange twists if you like.

NUTRITION AT A GLANCE
Per serving: 185 calories, 11 g fat, 8 g saturated fat, 13 g protein, 8 g carbohydrate, 1 g fiber, 144 mg sodium

Chocolate Meringue Kisses

MAKES 10 kisses (2 per serving)   **HANDS-ON TIME:** 30 minutes
TOTAL TIME: 1½ hours, including resting time

Don't be afraid to use a pastry bag. Once you get the hang of it, piping meringue is really easy. If you don't have one, just snip the corner off a resealable plastic bag and use that for piping. Unfilled, baked meringues keep for a week, tightly covered, at room temperature. Wait to sandwich the pairs together with the whipped topping until just before serving. Enjoy a couple of these with a glass of fat-free or 1% milk for a dessert "snack."

2 egg whites, at room temperature

¼ teaspoon cream of tartar

½ cup granular sugar substitute

2 tablespoons unsweetened cocoa powder

½ teaspoon vanilla extract

10 teaspoons no-sugar-added lite whipped topping

Heat the oven to 250°F. Line a baking sheet with parchment paper.

In a large bowl, with an electric mixer at high speed, beat the egg whites and cream of tartar until soft peaks form, about 5 minutes. Add the sugar substitute, 1 tablespoon at a time, beating until stiff peaks form. Do not underbeat. Whisk in the cocoa powder and vanilla until blended.

Fit a large star nozzle onto a pastry bag. Fill the pastry bag with the meringue. Pipe 20 meringues onto the baking sheet.

Bake for 30 minutes, or until the meringues are crisp and dry. Turn the oven off and let them cool in the oven for 30 minutes. Remove from the baking sheet.

Sandwich pairs of cooled meringues together with 1 teaspoon whipped topping to make a kiss.

NUTRITION AT A GLANCE
Per kiss: 18 calories, 0.2 g fat, 0 g saturated fat, 1 g protein, 3 g carbohydrate, 0 g fiber, 11 mg sodium

TIP: Make sure your mixing bowl is completely dry and clean of grease or the whites will not whip up enough.

Coconut Panna Cotta

MAKES 4 panna cotta **HANDS-ON TIME:** 15 minutes **TOTAL TIME:** 3 hours

Panna cotta, a popular Italian dessert, means "cooked cream." While heavy cream is typically used, we've used a combo of silky lite coconut milk and soy milk instead. The result is a cool, sweet, and extremely luscious dessert. You can make the panna cotta several days ahead, cover with plastic wrap, and refrigerate until ready to serve. This recipe can easily be doubled.

1 envelope unflavored gelatin

1½ cups unsweetened lite coconut milk

1 cup low-fat plain unsweetened soy milk

⅓ cup granular sugar substitute

½ teaspoon ground cinnamon

½ teaspoon vanilla extract

In a glass measuring cup, sprinkle the gelatin over ¼ cup cold water. Let stand for 5 minutes, or until softened. Place the measuring cup in a pan of simmering water and heat until the gelatin has dissolved, about 2 minutes.

In a large bowl, stir together the coconut milk, soy milk, sugar substitute, cinnamon, vanilla, and dissolved gelatin. Pour into four 8-ounce custard cups and refrigerate for at least 3 hours, or until set.

When ready to serve, run a butter knife or small spatula around the edge of each dessert and invert onto a serving plate.

NUTRITION AT A GLANCE
Per panna cotta: 111 calories, 7 g fat, 5 g saturated fat, 5 g protein, 6 g carbohydrate, 1 g fiber, 30 mg sodium

Lemon Buttermilk Sherbet

MAKES 8 (½-cup) servings   HANDS-ON TIME: 5 minutes   TOTAL TIME: 30 minutes plus chilling

A homemade frozen dessert is always a welcome ending to any meal, and this rich-tasting sherbet is a true treat for Phase 1 dieters. Here, agave nectar (see page 99) provides a natural alternative to granular sugar substitute.

2 cups light (1.5%) buttermilk

Grated zest of 2 lemons

3 tablespoons fresh lemon juice

⅔ cup light agave nectar

Lemon twists or fresh mint leaves, for garnish

In a large bowl, whisk together the buttermilk, lemon zest, lemon juice, and agave nectar. Transfer to an ice cream maker and process according to the manufacturer's instructions. Freeze until ready to serve, then garnish with lemon twists or mint leaves.

NUTRITION AT A GLANCE
Per serving: 106 calories, 0.5 g fat, 0.3 g saturated fat, 2 g protein, 25 g carbohydrate, 0 g fiber, 64 mg sodium

Variation: For a Phase 2 dessert, make Strawberry Buttermilk Sherbet: In a bowl, combine 1 package (15 ounces) thawed frozen strawberries (not in syrup) with the agave nectar. Let stand for 30 minutes. Transfer the mixture to a food processor and add the buttermilk and 2 tablespoons lemon juice. (Omit the lemon zest.) Purée until smooth and proceed with the recipe. Garnish with strawberries or raspberries. Makes 12 (½-cup) servings.

NUTRITION AT A GLANCE
Per serving: 82 calories, 0.4 g fat, 0.2 g saturated fat, 2 g protein, 20 g carbohydrate, 1 g fiber, 44 mg sodium

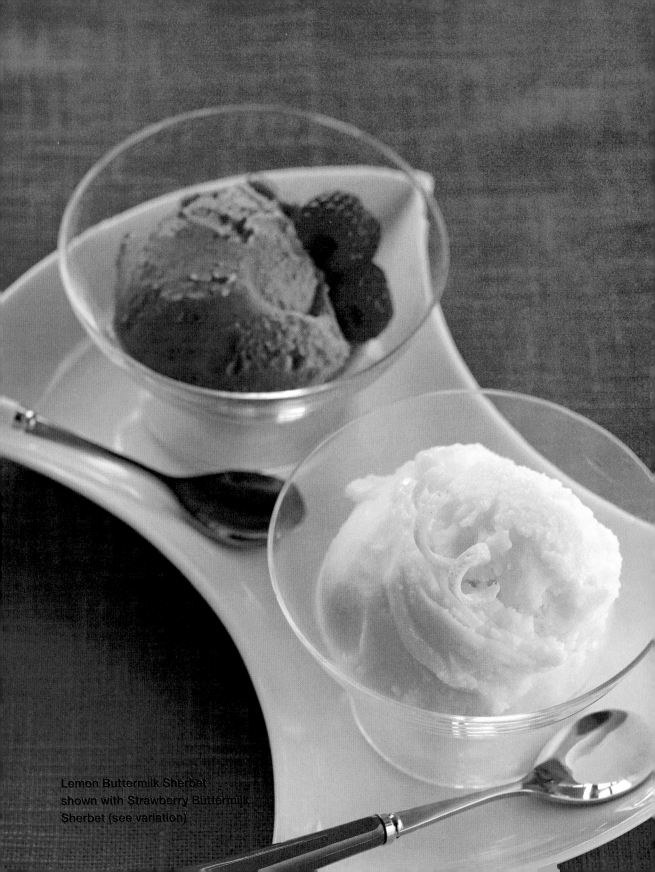

Lemon Buttermilk Sherbet
shown with Strawberry Buttermilk
Sherbet (see variation)

HOW TO EAT ON PHASE 1

On the following pages, you will find 2 weeks of sample meal plans for Phase 1, created in part with a number of delicious recipes from this book. Use these Meal Plans as is or as guidelines, making up your own menus as you see fit.

Keep in mind that the South Beach Diet doesn't require you to measure what you eat in ounces, calories, or anything else. Weighing, measuring, and counting are certainly not conducive to a pleasant lifestyle, and it is an approach to weight loss you're unlikely to sustain. Generally, if you are making the right food choices most of the time, portion control takes care of itself.

Your meals should be of normal size—enough to satisfy your hunger. And while you should never leave a meal hungry, that doesn't mean that you must clean your plate. Try to eat slowly so that your brain has time to detect your normal rise in blood sugar. This becomes much easier once you have completed a few days of of Phase 1 and any cravings you may have, especially for sweets, baked goods, and other refined carbohydrates, have largely disappeared. (See page 4 for more information on Phase 1.)

While we don't generally recommend weighing and measuring on the South Beach Diet, there are a few exceptions: We do suggest that you eat a minimum of 2 cups of vegetables with lunch and dinner so you get the maximum antioxidant and fiber benefits, and we also encourage you to work 2 cups of nonfat or low-fat dairy (including yogurt) into your diet each day. We also limit nuts to one serving per day and monounsaturated and polyunsaturated fats to 2 tablespoons a day. And of course we encourage you to drink water throughout the day to stay well hydrated.

DAY 1

BREAKFAST

6 ounces vegetable juice cocktail

Poached Egg Arrabiata (page 26)

3 slices Canadian bacon

Coffee or tea with 1% or fat-free milk and sugar substitute

MIDMORNING SNACK

1 reduced-fat spreadable cheese wedge with celery sticks

Mocha Frappé (page 56)

LUNCH

Clear mushroom beef soup (beef broth with reconstituted dried mushrooms)

Herbed Chicken and Bean Salad with Ranch Dressing (page 94)

MIDAFTERNOON SNACK

¼ cup (2 ounces) hummus with red, green, yellow, and/or orange bell pepper strips

DINNER

Chili-Rubbed Flank Steak with Sweet Onion Relish (page 181)

Quick Creamed Spinach (page 215)

Sliced tomatoes and Vidalia onion with 2 tablespoons low-sugar prepared dressing of your choice

DESSERT

Silken Chocolate Pudding (page 237)

DAY 2

BREAKFAST

6 ounces tomato juice

Mini Breakfast Frittatas (page 28)

Coffee or tea with 1% or fat-free milk and sugar substitute

MIDMORNING SNACK

Smoked Turkey Roll-Up with Lemony Avocado Spread (page 68)

LUNCH

"Tortilla" Soup (page 73)

Tex-Mex Steak Salad with Salsa Dressing (page 80)

MIDAFTERNOON SNACK

Mini red bell pepper halves with Spinach and Artichoke Dip (page 49)

DINNER

Baked Halibut with Asparagus and Shiitake Mushrooms (page 122)

Radicchio and endive salad with 2 tablespoons low-sugar prepared dressing of your choice

DESSERT

Almond-Jam Bars (page 247)

8 ounces fat-free or 1% milk

DAY 3

BREAKFAST

6 ounces vegetable juice cocktail

2 scrambled eggs with fresh herbs

2 slices turkey bacon

Jícama Hash Browns (page 223)

Coffee or tea with 1% or fat-free milk and sugar substitute

MIDMORNING SNACK

1 part-skim mozzarella cheese stick with radishes

LUNCH

California Turkey Salad with Fresh Tomato-Lime Dressing (page 81)

MIDAFTERNOON SNACK

Indian-style yogurt dip (mix ½ cup nonfat or low-fat plain yogurt with a little ground cumin, coriander, and turmeric)

Broccoli and cauliflower florets, for dipping

DINNER

Spicy Pork Skewers with Cashew Sauce (page 167)

Assorted grilled vegetables (asparagus, zucchini, bell peppers)

Bibb lettuce salad with 2 tablespoons red wine vinaigrette or low-sugar prepared dressing of your choice

DESSERT

Cannoli Pudding (page 233)

DAY 4

6 ounces tomato juice

Ham and reduced-fat cheese omelet with chives

Coffee or tea with 1% or fat-free milk and sugar substitute

1 reduced-fat extra-sharp Cheddar cheese stick with grape tomatoes

Two-Mushroom Cauliflower Soup (page 69)

Beef and Broccoli Salad with Mustard Vinaigrette (page 84)

Shrimp Cocktail with Creamy Chipotle Sauce (page 45)

Turkey Romesco (page 137)

Sautéed spinach with chopped shallots and fresh lemon juice

Red leaf lettuce salad with 2 tablespoons low-sugar prepared dressing of your choice

Black Bean Brownies (page 245)

8 ounces fat-free or 1% milk

DAY 5

BREAKFAST

6 ounces vegetable juice cocktail

South Beach Diet Breakfast Bowl (page 33)

Coffee or tea with 1% or fat-free milk and sugar substitute

MIDMORNING SNACK

½ cup fat-free (0%) Greek yogurt flavored with vanilla extract and sugar substitute

LUNCH

1 cup vegetable broth

Cajun Salmon and Arugula Salad (page 85)

Sugar-free gelatin

MIDAFTERNOON SNACK

Lettuce roll-up with 1 slice lean ham, 1 slice reduced-fat Swiss cheese, and Dijon mustard

DINNER

Mushroom-Beef Burger with Watercress Cream (page 178) on a bed of lettuce

Roasted asparagus spears with sea salt

Sliced beefsteak tomatoes sprinkled with sherry vinegar

DESSERT

Coconut-Almond Macaroons (page 236)

8 ounces fat-free or 1% milk

DAY 6

BREAKFAST

6 ounces tomato juice

Ham and Cheese Frico Breakwich (page 30)

Coffee or tea with 1% or fat-free milk and sugar substitute

MIDMORNING SNACK

Plum tomatoes topped with 1 ounce reduced-fat turkey pepperoni

Spiced Chai Tea Smoothie (page 59)

LUNCH

Picadillo-Style Lentil Stew (page 198)

Mesclun salad with 2 tablespoons low-sugar prepared dressing of your choice

MIDAFTERNOON SNACK

Smoked-Trout Deviled Eggs (page 51)

DINNER

Goat Cheese and Arugula–Stuffed Chicken Breast (page 156)

Warm Mushroom Salad with Toasted Pecans (page 209)

DESSERT

Chocolate-Meringue Kisses (page 264)

8 ounces fat-free or 1% milk

DAY 7

BREAKFAST

6 ounces vegetable juice cocktail

"Fried" Egg in Mushroom Cap (page 35)

Coffee or tea with 1% or fat-free milk and sugar substitute

MIDMORNING SNACK

Cherry tomatoes stuffed with reduced-fat cottage cheese

Latte with fat-free or 1% milk (sweetened with sugar substitute, if desired)

LUNCH

Quick Cobb Salad (page 93)

MIDAFTERNOON SNACK

Broccoli, Pepper, and Cheese Bites (page 41)

DINNER

Roasted Pecan Salmon with Lentil-Tomato Salad (page 108)

Roasted or steamed green beans with chopped fresh mint

DESSERT

Lemon Buttermilk Sherbet (page 266)

DAY 8

BREAKFAST

6 ounces tomato juice

Omelet with artichoke hearts and baby spinach

2 slices turkey bacon

Coffee or tea with 1% or fat-free milk and sugar substitute

MIDMORNING SNACK

1 ounce reduced-fat Gouda cheese with celery sticks

LUNCH

Chicken Salad Niçoise (page 97)

MIDAFTERNOON SNACK

½ cup fat-free black bean dip with assorted bell pepper slices

DINNER

Lemon-Dill Soup with Scallops (page 64)

Eggplant Caprese (page 186)

Summer Salad with Fresh Herb Vinaigrette (page 214)

DESSERT

Coconut Panna Cotta (page 265)

DAY 9

BREAKFAST

6 ounces vegetable juice cocktail

Eggs Florentine (2 poached eggs on a bed of spinach sautéed in extra-virgin olive oil)

Coffee or tea with 1% or fat-free milk and sugar substitute

MIDMORNING SNACK

Smoked salmon on cucumber rounds

LUNCH

Clear broth

Double-Soy Salad (page 99)

Sugar-free gelatin

MIDAFTERNOON SNACK

½ cup reduced-fat cottage cheese with chopped green bell pepper in a red bell pepper "cup"

DINNER

Chicken with Cremini Cream Sauce (page 140)

Roasted Green and Wax Beans with Walnuts (page 211)

DESSERT

No-sugar-added Fudgsicle

8 ounces fat-free or 1% milk

DAY 10

BREAKFAST

6 ounces tomato juice

2 eggs scrambled with chopped onion and jarred roasted red peppers

3 slices Canadian bacon

Coffee or tea with 1% or fat-free milk and sugar substitute

MIDMORNING SNACK

Lettuce roll-up with 1 slice lean deli roast beef, 1 slice Provolone, and horseradish sauce

Mocha Frappé (page 56)

LUNCH

White Bean and Escarole Soup with Shaved Parmesan (page 62)

MIDAFTERNOON SNACK

Caprese bites (cut 1 part-skim mozzarella stick into 4 pieces; place each piece in a hollowed-out cherry tomato and microwave to melt cheese, if desired)

DINNER

Grouper with Salsa Verde (page 128)

Baby Greens and Grilled Asparagus with Shallot Vinaigrette (page 224)

DESSERT

Peanut butter delight (in a blender, process ½ cup part-skim ricotta, 1 tablespoon natural peanut butter, ½ teaspoon pure vanilla extract, and 1 packet granular sugar substitute until smooth; chill and serve)

DAY 11

BREAKFAST

6 ounces vegetable juice cocktail

1 cup fat-free (0%) Greek yogurt and 15 pistachios

Coffee or tea with 1% or fat-free milk and sugar substitute

MIDMORNING SNACK

1 ounce reduced-fat Cheddar cheese cubes with chilled steamed asparagus spears

LUNCH

Chunky Gazpacho Salad with Grilled Scallops (page 101)

Sugar-free gelatin

MIDAFTERNOON SNACK

Lettuce roll-up with 1 slice smoked turkey, 1 slice avocado, and 1 slice reduced-fat pepper Jack cheese

DINNER

Satay Chicken Burger (page 152)

Sautéed snow peas and water chestnuts

Tossed salad of mixed baby greens with 2 tablespoons low-sugar prepared dressing of your choice

DESSERT

Vanilla chill (blend 1 cup nonfat or low-fat plain yogurt, ⅔ cup low-fat plain or artificially sweetened soymilk, 1 teaspoon pure vanilla extract, ice cubes, and a sprinkling of cinnamon)

DAY 12

BREAKFAST

6 ounces tomato juice

Asparagus and Red Pepper Frittata with Goat Cheese (page 193)

Coffee or tea with 1% or fat-free milk and sugar substitute

MIDMORNING SNACK

½ cup baba ghannouj with assorted bell pepper strips

LUNCH

"Tortilla" Soup (page 73)

Speedy Fajita Salad (page 100)

MIDAFTERNOON SNACK

½ cup roasted canned garbanzo beans sprinkled with black pepper

DINNER

Striped Bass Roasted with Cauliflower, Lemon, and Olives (page 109)

Fennel, Cucumber, and Watercress Salad (page 219)

DESSERT

Mocha ricotta crème (whisk together ½ cup part-skim ricotta cheese,
¼ teaspoon pure vanilla extract, 1 packet granular sugar substitute,
½ teaspoon unsweetened cocoa powder)

DAY 13

BREAKFAST

6 ounces vegetable juice cocktail

Egg white omelet with chopped Canadian bacon and mushrooms

Coffee or tea with 1% or fat-free milk and sugar substitute

MIDMORNING SNACK

1 reduced-fat French onion or garlic spreadable cheese wedge
in endive leaves

LUNCH

Spinach and Bean Salad with Shrimp (page 105)

MIDAFTERNOON SNACK

½ cup reduced-fat cottage cheese with slivered almonds

DINNER

Grilled Sirloin Steak with Shallot-Mustard Sauce (page 168)

Roasted cherry tomatoes with fresh dill

Cucumber salad with 2 tablespoons low-sugar prepared dressing
of your choice

DESSERT

½ cup fat-free (0%) Greek yogurt flavored with pure vanilla extra

Chocolate Meringue Kisses (page 264)

DAY 14

BREAKFAST

6 ounces tomato juice

Energy shake (in a blender, combine 1 cup artificially sweetened vanilla low-fat soy milk, ½ cup low-fat plain yogurt, ¼ cup silken tofu, and 6 almonds; blend until smooth)

3 slices Canadian bacon

Coffee or tea with 1% or fat-free milk and sugar substitute

MIDMORNING SNACK

5 part-skim mozzarella balls with grape tomatoes

LUNCH

Buffalo Chicken Salad (page 104)

Sugar-free gelatin

MIDAFTERNOON SNACK

1 ounce feta cheese cubes marinated in 2 tablespoons lemon vinaigrette

DINNER

Loin Lamb Chops with Mint Pesto (page 166)

Cauliflower purée

Roasted eggplant slices with chopped kalamata olives and chopped tomatoes

DESSERT

Maple ricotta crème (ricotta cheese drizzled with sugar-free maple syrup)

HOW TO EAT ON PHASE 2

On the following pages, you'll find 2 weeks of sample Meal Plans for Phase 2, which use a number of recipes from this book. As with Phase 1, feel free to use these Meal Plans as guidelines and make up your own plans as you see fit.

The key to continuing your weight loss success on Phase 2 is to gradually reintroduce foods that were off limits on Phase 1, so you can better monitor your hunger and possible cravings. For example, you can begin Phase 2 by having one whole-grain food and one fruit each day for the first few days in addition to your lean protein, vegetables, and low-fat dairy. If you continue to lose weight, you can gradually add more fruits, whole grains, and other foods. You will continue Phase 2 until you reach a weight that's healthy for you. Remember that this is a slower weight-loss phase than Phase 1: Losing 1 to 2 pounds a week on Phase 2 is excellent. (See page 4 for more information on Phase 2.)

As with Phase 1, continue to eat plenty of vegetables, enjoy 2 to 3 cups of low-fat or nonfat dairy each day, and be sure to drink water throughout the day to stay hydrated.

A note about whole grains: On Phase 2, you will be introducing whole grains into your diet, but be sure you purchase the right ones. When you buy whole-grain breads and other products, be sure the label says "100% whole wheat" or "whole grain," not "enriched" or "fortified" grain or simply "100% wheat." The process of refining white flour depletes it of much of its fiber and nutrients.

DAY 1

BREAKFAST

6 ounces vegetable juice cocktail

Overnight Oatmeal (page 250)

2 scrambled eggs with chopped tomato and tarragon

2 slices turkey bacon

Coffee or tea with 1% or fat-free milk and sugar substitute

MIDMORNING SNACK

1 ounce reduced-fat Cheddar cheese cubes

Grape or cherry tomatoes

LUNCH

Chicken or beef broth with sliced scallions

Jalapeño Shrimp Salad (page 90)

MIDAFTERNOON SNACK

Spicy Lemon Edamame (page 52)

Spiced Chai Tea Smoothie (page 59)

DINNER

Five-Spice Grilled Chicken with Asian Dipping Sauce (page 163)

Broccoli stir-fry (in a wok, toss broccoli florets with chopped garlic and ginger and some reduced-sodium soy sauce, a little sesame oil, and dry sherry)

DESSERT

Strawberry Fool (page 241)

DAY 2

BREAKFAST

6 ounces tomato juice

Ham and feta cheese omelet with chives

Coffee or tea with 1% or fat-free milk and sugar substitute

MIDMORNING SNACK

½ cup fat-free (0%) Greek yogurt with pure vanilla extract and granular sugar substitute

LUNCH

Italian Tuna Burger (page 133)

Sliced tomatoes and lettuce leaves, for topping burger

MIDAFTERNOON SNACK

Ginger Chicken Salad in Cucumber Cups (page 40)

DINNER

Pork Tenderloin "Steak" with Prunes (page 183)

Steamed broccoli with fresh lemon juice

DESSERT

Dark Chocolate Bark with Walnuts (page 242)

DAY 3

BREAKFAST

6 ounces vegetable juice cocktail

"Fried" Egg in Mushroom Cap (page 35)

3 slices Canadian bacon

Coffee or tea with 1% or fat-free milk and sugar substitute

MIDMORNING SNACK

¼ cup Roasted Adobo Lentils (page 54)

LUNCH

Asparagus Bisque (page 67)

Open-Face Stack Sandwich (page 74)

MIDAFTERNOON SNACK

Broccoli, Pepper, and Cheese Bites (page 41)

DINNER

Lemony Stuffed Mushrooms (page 44)

Flank Steak with Chimichurri (page 175)

Cauliflower purée with roasted garlic

Chicory and tomato salad with 2 tablespoons low-sugar ranch dressing or other low-sugar prepared dressing of your choice

DESSERT

Glazed Bananas with Lime Cream (page 234)

DAY 4

BREAKFAST

6 ounces tomato juice

Tofu, Spinach, and Egg Scramble (page 29)

Coffee or tea with 1% or fat-free milk and sugar substitute

MIDMORNING SNACK

Hollowed-out plum tomatoes stuffed with fresh part-skim mozzarella

LUNCH

Shrimp Cone (page 71)

Jícama and radish salad

MIDAFTERNOON SNACK

Cucumber slices topped with 2 tablespoons reduced-fat herb-flavored
cream cheese

DINNER

Chicken Tri-Colore (page 158)

Braised Balsamic Carrots (page 210)

Arugula, Frisée, and Roasted Pear Salad (page 217)

DESSERT

Cannoli Pudding (page 233)

DAY 5

6 ounces vegetable juice cocktail

Fruit and Yogurt Breakfast Parfait (page 25)

Coffee or tea with 1% or fat-free milk and sugar substitute

Smoked-Trout Deviled Eggs (page 51)

"Tortilla" Soup (page 73)

Inside-Out Cheeseburger (page 147)

¼ cup (2 ounces) hummus with jarred roasted red peppers

Mussels and Leeks in Fennel Broth (page 119)

Seven-Vegetable Salad (page 82)

Black Bean Brownies (page 245)

8 ounces fat-free or 1% milk

DAY 6

BREAKFAST

6 ounces tomato juice

Ham and Cheese Frico Breakwich (page 30)

Coffee or tea with 1% or fat-free milk and sugar substitute

MIDMORNING SNACK

½ cup fat-free (0%) Greek yogurt with chopped veggies

LUNCH

Asian Roast Pork Salad (page 102)

MIDAFTERNOON SNACK

Smoked Turkey Roll-Up with Lemony Avocado Spread (page 68)

DINNER

Coconut Shrimp Curry (page 130)

½ cup cooked quick-cooking barley or brown rice

Sliced cucumber and red onion salad with 2 tablespoons sherry vinaigrette or low-sugar prepared dressing of your choice

DESSERT

Chocolate Meringue Kisses (page 264)

8 ounces fat-free or 1% milk

DAY 7

BREAKFAST

6 ounces vegetable juice cocktail

Poached Egg Arrabbiata (page 26)

3 slices Canadian bacon

Coffee or tea with 1% or fat-free milk and sugar substitute

MIDMORNING SNACK

1 ounce reduced-fat Cheddar cheese cubes

Spiced Chai Tea Smoothie (page 59)

LUNCH

Lemon-Caper Chicken (page 155)

Roasted Green and Wax Beans with Walnuts (page 211)

MIDAFTERNOON SNACK

½ cup baba ghannouj

DINNER

Pan-Grilled Duck Breast with Orange Salsa (page 143)

Oven roasted zucchini and yellow squash with shaved Parmesan

DESSERT

Fresh sliced pear with pomegranate seeds and a dollop of reduced-fat sour cream

DAY 8

BREAKFAST

6 ounces tomato juice

1 cup fat-free (0%) yogurt with pure vanilla extract

Apricot-Oat Bar (page 36)

Coffee or tea with 1% or fat-free milk and sugar substitute

MIDMORNING SNACK

2 deviled egg halves

LUNCH

Pork and Pepper Stew (page 176)

MIDAFTERNOON SNACK

¼ cup (2 ounces) hummus with crudités

DINNER

Spinach and Four-Cheese Lasagna (page 257)

Sliced tomato salad with 2 tablespoons no-sugar-added prepared dressing of your choice

DESSERT

Silken Chocolate Pudding (page 237)

DAY 9

BREAKFAST

½ grapefruit

2 scrambled eggs with chopped ham and chives

Jícama Hash Browns (page 223)

Coffee or tea with 1% or fat-free milk and sugar substitute

MIDMORNING SNACK

½ cup fat-free (0%) Greek yogurt with ¼ cup chopped cashews

LUNCH

Grilled Summer Squash Pizzette (page 63)

Arugula salad with fresh lemon juice and freshly ground black pepper

MIDAFTERNOON SNACK

½ cup fat-free black bean dip with veggie dippers

DINNER

Quick Turkey Tagine (page 150)

Lemon Quinoa Salad (page 220)

DESSERT

Lemon Buttermilk Sherbet (page 266)

DAY 10

BREAKFAST

6 ounces vegetable juice cocktail

Fluffy Berry-Studded Pancakes (page 37)

Coffee or tea with 1% or fat-free milk and sugar substitute

MIDMORNING SNACK

1 hard-boiled egg with bell pepper strips

Mocha Frappé (page 56)

LUNCH

Crispy Tofu with Broccolini (page 201)

MIDAFTERNOON SNACK

1 Granny Smith apple with 2 tablespoons natural no-sugar-added
peanut butter

DINNER

Shrimp Scampi with Whole-Wheat Pasta (page 111)

Summer Salad with Fresh Herb Vinaigrette (page 214)

DESSERT

Chocolate Truffle Tartlets (page 232)

DAY 11

BREAKFAST

Cantaloupe wedge with a squeeze of fresh lime

Mini Breakfast Frittatas (page 28)

3 slices Canadian bacon

Coffee or tea with 1% or fat-free milk and sugar substitute

MIDMORNING SNACK

1 wedge reduced-fat French onion spreadable cheese with carrot sticks

LUNCH

Spiced Sweet Potato–Tomato Soup (page 76)

Mini Turkey Meatloaf (page 141)

Tossed green salad with 2 tablespoons balsamic vinaigrette or low-sugar prepared dressing of your choice

MIDAFTERNOON SNACK

½ cup South Beach Diet Snack Mix (page 55)

DINNER

Beef Burgundy

Endive salad with 2 tablespoons low-sugar prepared dressing of your choice

DESSERT

Mini Apple Tarts (page 240)

DAY 12

BREAKFAST

6 ounces tomato juice

2 scrambled eggs with shredded reduced-fat Cheddar cheese

Lemon-Raspberry Muffin (page 32)

Coffee or tea with 1% or fat-free milk and sugar substitute

MIDMORNING SNACK

½ cup fat-free (0%) Greek yogurt with 15 pistachios

LUNCH

Confetti Crab Salad (page 87)

MIDAFTERNOON SNACK

Triple Berry Cooler (page 58)

DINNER

Chicken with Wine-Braised Mushrooms (page 157)

½ cup whole wheat couscous

Sautéed Swiss chard

DESSERT

Grilled Summer Fruit (page 244)

DAY 13

BREAKFAST

6 ounces vegetable juice cocktail

Multigrain Toaster Waffles (page 251)

2 slices turkey bacon

Coffee or tea with 1% or fat-free milk and sugar substitute

MIDMORNING SNACK

½ cup nonfat or low-fat plain yogurt with chopped cucumbers and peppers

LUNCH

White Chipotle Chicken Chili (page 255)

Hearts of romaine with 2 tablespoons low-sugar prepared dressing of your choice

MIDAFTERNOON SNACK

Red Delicious apple with 1 ounce sliced reduced-fat cheese

DINNER

Red Snapper Veracruz (page 127)

Roasted Green and Wax Beans, no walnuts (page 211)

DESSERT

Orange-Almond Ricotta Cheesecake (page 263)

DAY 14

BREAKFAST

6 ounces tomato juice

Almond French Toast with Warm Blueberry Syrup (page 24)

3 slices Canadian bacon

Coffee or tea with 1% or fat-free milk and sugar substitute

MIDMORNING SNACK

1 part-skim mozzarella cheese stick

LUNCH

Vegetable Tart (page 256)

MIDAFTERNOON SNACK

¼ cup Roasted Adobo Lentils (page 54)

DINNER

Grilled Tandoori Chicken (page 259)

Cucumber-Mint Raita (page 229)

Indian-Spiced Mashed Sweet Potatoes (page 218)

DESSERT

Apricot-Berry Dessert Pizza (page 239)

INDEX

Underscored page references indicate boxed text. **Boldface** references indicate photographs.

VISIT SOUTHBEACHDIET.COM

For more great recipes, plus customized Meal Plans, weight-loss tools, and support from registered dietitians and a vibrant community of South Beach Diet followers, visit www.SouthBeachDiet.com.

Conversion Chart

These equivalents have been slightly rounded to make measuring easier.

Volume Measurements

U.S.	Imperial	Metric
¼ tsp	–	1 ml
½ tsp	–	2 ml
1 tsp	–	5 ml
1 Tbsp	–	15 ml
2 Tbsp (1 oz)	1 fl oz	30 ml
¼ cup (2 oz)	2 fl oz	60 ml
⅓ cup (3 oz)	3 fl oz	80 ml
½ cup (4 oz)	4 fl oz	120 ml
⅔ cup (5 oz)	5 fl oz	160 ml
¾ cup (6 oz)	6 fl oz	180 ml
1 cup (8 oz)	8 fl oz	240 ml

Weight Measurements

U.S.	Metric
1 oz	30 g
2 oz	60 g
4 oz (¼ lb)	115 g
5 oz (⅓ lb)	145 g
6 oz	170 g
7 oz	200 g
8 oz (½ lb)	230 g
10 oz	285 g
12 oz (¾ lb)	340 g
14 oz	400 g
16 oz (1 lb)	455 g
2.2 lb	1 kg

Length Measurements

U.S.	Metric
¼"	0.6 cm
½"	1.25 cm
1"	2.5 cm
2"	5 cm
4"	11 cm
6"	15 cm
8"	20 cm
10"	25 cm
12" (1')	30 cm

Pan Sizes

U.S.	Metric
8" cake pan	20 × 4 cm sandwich or cake tin
9" cake pan	23 × 3.5 cm sandwich or cake tin
11" × 7" baking pan	28 × 18 cm baking tin
13" × 9" baking pan	32.5 × 23 cm baking tin
15" × 10" baking pan	38 × 25.5 cm baking tin (Swiss roll tin)
1½ qt baking dish	1.5 liter baking dish
2 qt baking dish	2 liter baking dish
2 qt rectangular baking dish	30 × 19 cm baking dish
9" pie plate	22 × 4 or 23 × 4 cm pie plate
7" or 8" springform pan	18 or 20 cm springform or loose-bottom cake tin
9" × 5" loaf pan	23 × 13 cm or 2 lb narrow loaf tin or pâté tin

Temperatures

Fahrenheit	Centigrade	Gas
140°	60°	–
160°	70°	–
180°	80°	–
225°	105°	¼
250°	120°	½
275°	135°	1
300°	150°	2
325°	160°	3
350°	180°	4
375°	190°	5
400°	200°	6
425°	220°	7
450°	230°	8
475°	245°	9
500°	260°	–